Visual Guide for Clinicians
BREAST CANCER

Visual Guide for Clinicians

BREAST CANCER

Matthew D Barber
BSc (Hons), MBChB (Hons), MD, FRCS (Gen Surg)
Consultant Breast Surgeon
Edinburgh Breast Unit
Western General Hospital
Edinburgh, UK

Jeremy St J Thomas
MA, MRCS, MBBS (Hons), MRCP (UK), FRCPath
Consultant Pathologist
Department of Pathology
Western General Hospital
Edinburgh, UK

J Michael Dixon
BSc (Hons), MBChB, MD, FRCS (Edinburgh), FRCS (England), FRCP (Edin)
Consultant Surgeon and Professor of Surgery
Edinburgh Breast Unit
Clinical Director
Breakthrough Research Unit
Western General Hospital
Edinburgh, UK

CLINICAL PUBLISHING

OXFORD

Clinical Publishing
an imprint of Atlas Medical Publishing Ltd
Oxford Centre for Innovation
Mill Street, Oxford OX2 0JX, UK

Tel: +44 1865 811116
Fax: +44 1865 251550
Email: info@clinicalpublishing.co.uk
Web: www.clinicalpublishing.co.uk

Distributed in USA and Canada by:
Clinical Publishing
30 Amberwood Parkway
Ashland, OH 44805, USA

Tel: 800-247-6553 (toll free within US and Canada)
Fax: 419-281-6883
Email: order@bookmasters.com

Distributed in UK and Rest of World by:
Marston Book Services Ltd
PO Box 269
Abingdon
Oxon OX14 4YN, UK

Tel: +44 1235 465500
Fax: +44 1235 465555
Email: trade.orders@marston.co.uk

ISBN 978 1 84692 093 6
e-ISBN 978 1 84692 636 5

The publisher makes no representation, express or implied, that the dosages in this book are correct. Readers must therefore always check the product information and clinical procedures with the most up-to-date published product information and data sheets provided by the manufacturers and the most recent codes of conduct and safety regulations. The authors and the publisher do not accept any liability for any errors in the text or for the misuse or misapplication of material in this work.

Printed by Marston Book Services Ltd, Abingdon, Oxon, UK

Contents

Abbreviations

ADH atypical ductal hyperplasia
ALH atypical lobular hyperplasia
CC craniocaudal (view)
CI confidence interval
CT computed tomography
DCIS ductal carcinoma *in situ*
ER oestrogen receptor
FISH fluorescence *in situ* hybridization
FNA fine needle aspiration
G-CSF granulocyte-colony stimulating factor
H&E haematoxylin and eosin

HER human epidermal growth factor receptor
HRT hormone replacement therapy
LCIS lobular carcinoma *in situ*
LHRH luteinizing hormone releasing hormone
MLO mediolateral oblique (view)
MRI magnetic resonance imaging
NST no special type
OS overall survival
PAP papanicolau
PET positron emission tomography
PGR progesterone receptor

Acknowledgements

Thanks to Carolyn Beveridge, Yvette Godwin, Isobel Arnott, Frances Yuille, Cameron Raine, Larry Hayward, St John's Hospital Medical Photography Department, St John's Hospital and Western General Hospital Multidisciplinary Breast teams, and especially to the patients for their assistance in the preparation of this book.

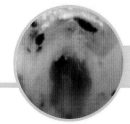
Chapter 1

Anatomy, Physiology, Symptom Assessment, and Epidemiology

ANATOMY AND PHYSIOLOGY

Breast (Figures 1.1, 1.2)

The mammary gland is a distinguishing feature of mammals and its primary role is to produce milk to nourish offspring. In humans, the breast has a multitude of further roles including being a major female sexual characteristic and a key part of female body image.

The breast develops within the superficial fascia of the anterior chest wall. Prior to puberty, both in men and women, the breast consists only of a few ducts within a connective tissue stroma. True breast development (thelarche) begins in females at puberty around the age of 10 years under the influence of oestrogen and progesterone. The breast is hemispherical in shape with an extension towards the axilla and becomes more pendulous with age. It extends from around the level of the second rib to seventh rib in the midclavicular line and from the lateral edge of the sternum to the midaxillary line. It overlies the pectoralis major, serratus anterior, and rectus abdominis muscles. Strands of fibrous connective tissue (Cooper's ligaments) run from the skin overlying the breast to the underlying chest wall providing a supportive framework.

The breast contains 12–15 major breast ducts which drain to the nipple, connected to a series of branching ducts ending in the terminal duct lobular unit, the functional milk-producing unit of the breast. Breast ducts are lined by a layer of cuboidal cells surrounded by a network of myoepithelial cells supported by connective tissue stroma, and are embedded in a variable amount of fat. The major subareolar breast ducts open on the surface of the nipple, which protrudes from the breast surface. The nipple and surrounding areola are variably pigmented and their skin is rich in smooth muscle fibres.

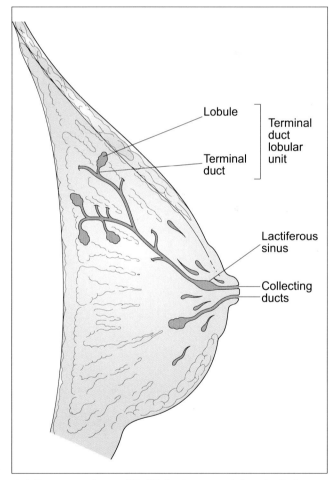

1.1 Breast anatomy. 12–15 ducts open at the nipple from the ductal system of the breast, which originates in the milk-producing functional unit – the terminal duct lobular unit.

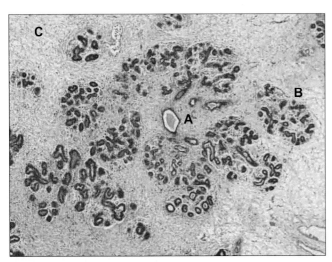

1.2 Normal adult breast during reproductive years: photomicrograph shows a complete terminal duct lobular unit. A, terminal duct; B, lobules; C, surrounding nonspecialized stroma.

During pregnancy, the terminal duct lobular units proliferate under the influence of increased levels of oestrogen, progesterone, and prolactin. Milk is produced as a result of secretion of prolactin and oxytocin from the pituitary in response to suckling.

Fluctuations in oestrogen and progesterone concentrations prior to and following the menopause result in atrophic changes to the glandular and connective tissue components of the breast.

The nerve supply of the breast is in a segmental pattern from the intercostal nerves and the blood supply is derived from branches of the internal mammary, lateral thoracic, and pectoral vessels.

Lymphatics (Figure 1.3)

The lymphatic drainage of the breast is of great clinical importance. About 5% of lymph from the breast drains medially through the intercostal spaces to nodes alongside the internal mammary vessels. The remaining 95% drains towards the axilla in one or two larger channels. Only a small amount of lymph drains through the pectoral and rectus fascia or to the opposite breast. The 20–30 axillary lymph nodes which receive the majority of lymph from the breast are conveniently classified according to their relationship with the pectoralis minor muscle into three levels: level 1 nodes lie lateral to the muscle, level 2 behind, and level 3 medial.

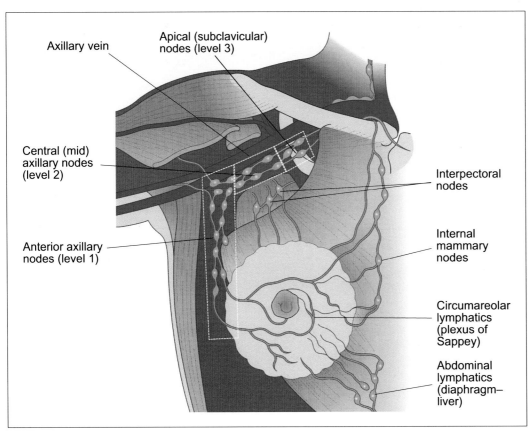

1.3 Lymphatic anatomy. The vast majority of lymph from the breast drains to the axilla. The axilla is divided into three levels: 1: lateral to pectoralis minor, 2: deep to pectoralis minor, and 3: medial to pectoralis minor.

Axilla (Figures 1.4, 1.5)

All patients with invasive breast cancer should undergo some form of axillary surgery to assess whether there is lymph node involvement. Knowledge of the anatomy of this area is crucial. The axilla is a pyramidal compartment between the arm and chest wall. The base is formed by axillary fascia and skin. The apex runs into the posterior triangle of the neck between the clavicle, first rib, and scapula. The pectoral muscles form the anterior wall and the serratus anterior muscle over the chest wall forms the medial wall. The posterior wall is formed by the subscapularis, teres major, and latissimus dorsi muscles and the lateral wall by the humerus. The axillary vein marks the superior boundary of routine axillary surgery with the axillary artery and brachial plexus lying above this. Several unnamed vessels are encountered in

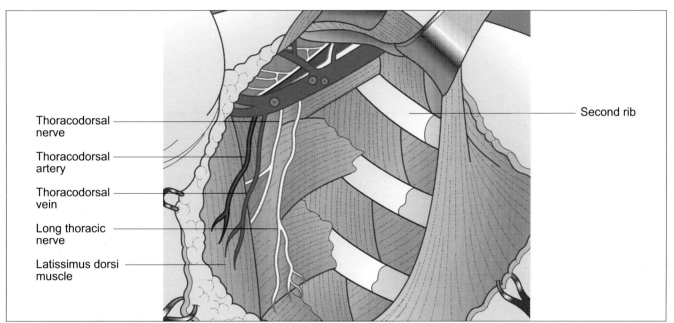

1.4 Axillary anatomy. The medial wall of the axilla is formed by the ribs and chest wall muscles, notably serratus anterior over which runs the long thoracic nerve. Posteriorly lie the subscapularis, teres major, and latissimus dorsi muscles over which run the thoracodorsal pedicle. The pectoral muscles lie anteriorly.

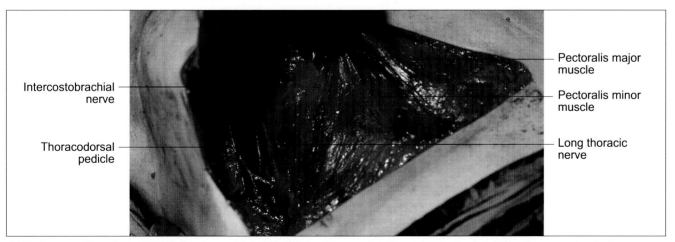

1.5 Intraoperative photograph following axillary clearance. The pectoralis major and minor muscles are retracted upwards. The long thoracic nerve is seen running along the chest wall. The thoracodoral pedicle runs at the back of the wound and an intercostobrachial nerve is seen running across the axillary space.

the anterior part of the axilla. The thoracodorsal artery and vein run from the subscapular vessels (from the third part of the axillary vessels) and the thoracodorsal nerve (arising from the posterior cord of the brachial plexus) emerges from below the axillary vein to run with the vessels over the subscapularis muscle towards the latissimus dorsi muscle. The long thoracic nerve arises from the upper roots of the brachial plexus to run down the chest wall over the serratus anterior muscle which it supplies. Two or three intercostobrachial nerves emerge from the chest wall and traverse the axilla to provide sensory supply to the skin of the axilla and upper inner arm.

ASSESSMENT OF THE BREAST

Triple assessment

Triple assessment is the combination of clinical, radiological, and pathological evaluation of a breast lesion (*Table 1.1*). Triple assessment should be used in all patients with a suspected breast lump and may be relevant in those with other symptoms. Imaging assessment consists of mammography (in those aged 35 years or over), and ultrasonography is recommended for all palpable and significant radiological abnormalities (at any age). Histological assessment usually involves core biopsy and/or fine needle aspiration (FNA) cytology. This combination of techniques increases the reliability of determining the cause of a clinical or image-detected abnormality (*Tables 1.2, 1.3*). It is

Table 1.1 Scoring system for triple assessment

1 Normal (or inadequate cytology)
2 Benign (or normal cytology)
3 Suspicious but probably benign
4 Suspicious and probably malignant
5 Malignant

recommended that all elements of the assessment process are reported on a scale of 1–5 with increasing concern of malignancy. In a patient with a discrete breast mass or abnormality seen on imaging, most centres offer immediate reporting of imaging and cytology of fine needle aspirates or touch preparation cytology from a core biopsy. 'One stop' clinics have advantages for women with benign lumps who can be reassured and discharged after a single visit and can allow rapid diagnosis in those with cancer.

Clinical history

A history is taken from the patient of the duration and nature of presenting symptoms. Further specific details of individual symptoms are of value and are outlined below. Past personal or familial breast problems should be elucidated. General factors such as past medical history, drugs, and allergies should be recorded. Hormonal risk factors for cancer such as age of menarche and menopause, parity, age of first birth,

Table 1.2 Accuracy of investigations in symptomatic breast clinic

	Clinical examination	Mammography	Ultrasonography	Fine needle aspiration cytology*	Core biopsy*
Sensitivity for cancer	86%	86%	90%	95%	85–98%
Sensitivity for benign disease	90%	90%	92%	95%	95%
Positive predictive value for cancer	95%	95%	95%	99.8%	100%

Sensitivity includes assessment as malignant and probably malignant
Accuracy of mammography varies with age
*Accuracy of biopsy techniques is improved by image guidance

Table 1.3 Symptoms and cancer risk in those attending a symptomatic clinic

	% of referrals	% with cancer	% of cancers
Lump	63.8	16.6	80.5
Pain	17.1	4.2	5.1
Nipple discharge	4.4	5.4	1.7
Change in shape	2.5	38.1	6.8

breast feeding, oral contraceptive or hormone replacement therapy use are traditionally documented, although they are of no value in achieving a diagnosis in an individual case. The history and examination findings should be recorded legibly and contemporaneously in the medical records, often on a standard form.

Clinical examination (Figures 1.6–1.9)

Breast examination should be conducted in a good light with the patient stripped to the waist in the presence of a chaperone. Initial examination is by inspection with the patient in the sitting position with hands by her side, paying particular attention to symmetry, nipple inversion, skin changes, and alterations in breast contour. The breast should also be inspected both with arms raised and with the chest wall muscles tensed and changes in the dynamic setting noted.

Palpation of the breasts is best performed in the supine position with the head supported and the arms above the head. Putting the hands above the head spreads the breast out over the chest wall and reduces the depth of breast tissue between the examiner's hands and the chest wall, and makes abnormal areas much easier to detect and define. All the breast tissue is examined using the most sensitive part of the hand, the fingertips. If an abnormality is identified, then it should be assessed for contour, texture, and any deep fixation by tensing the pectoralis major. All palpable lesions should be measured with callipers.

If there is a history of nipple discharge, the nipple should be gently squeezed to determine whether a pathological discharge is present. Careful note should be taken of whether discharge is emerging from single or multiple ducts and whether blood is present either frankly or on dipstick testing.

All women complaining of breast pain or tenderness should be examined for tenderness of the chest wall. With the patient in the sitting position, the hand may be pushed

Inspection

Palpation

1.6 The breasts are inspected with the patient seated and the arms raised and lowered and with the pectoral muscles tensed. The breasts are palpated in a systematic manner using the fingertips with the patient supine and with the head supported.

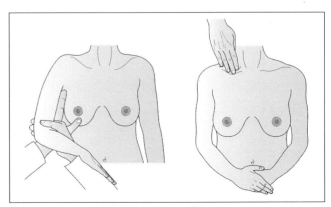

1.7 The axilla is examined with the patient sitting and their arm supported. The supraclavicular fossa is best examined from behind.

up behind the breast from below with pressure on the chest wall. The patient may also be rolled onto their side, allowing the breast to fall medially, exposing the edge of the pectoral muscle to palpation. The patient should be asked to indicate if there is any localized tenderness on palpation of the chest wall, and whether any discomfort evident during examination is similar to the pain they normally experience. Allowing the woman herself to confirm that the site of maximal tenderness is in the underlying chest wall rather than the breast is effective in reassuring patients that there is no significant breast problem.

The axilla is best examined with the patient sitting. The examiner's ipsilateral arm supports the patient's arm while the examiner's contralateral hand is placed high in the axilla on the chest wall and run carefully downwards. The supraclavicular fossa is examined from behind with the patient in a sitting position. A general examination of the cardiovascular and respiratory systems is useful in those in whom surgery is contemplated. If metastatic disease is suspected, then examination for bony tenderness, hepatomegaly, and pleural effusion may be valuable.

Imaging

Mammography (Figures 1.10–1.13)
Mammography requires compression of the breast between two plates and is uncomfortable. Two views (oblique and craniocaudal) of each breast are taken. A dose of less than 1.5 mGy is standard. Mammography allows detection of mass lesions, areas of parenchymal distortion, and microcalcifications. Breasts are relatively radiodense in younger women and thus mammography is not normally performed in those aged under 35 years. All patients with a breast cancer, regardless of age, should have mammography prior to surgery as it is valuable in assessing extent of disease. The introduction of digital technology offers opportunities in image manipulation, storage, and transmission. It may increase specificity in older women and increase sensitivity in younger women, although cost and fragility of equipment are concerns, particularly for mobile screening units.

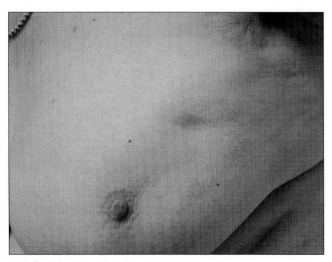

1.8 Inflammatory left breast cancer with swelling, oedema (*peau d'orange*), erythema, and nipple inversion. The lump of the underlying breast cancer can be difficult to feel in such circumstances.

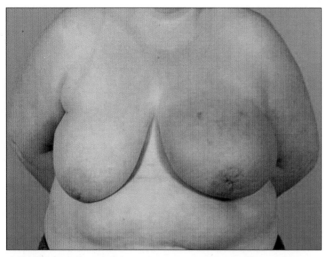

1.9 Subtle skin dimpling in the upper outer quadrant due to underlying breast cancer. Such dimpling is not due to direct skin involvement but to tethering of the connective tissue framework of the breast.

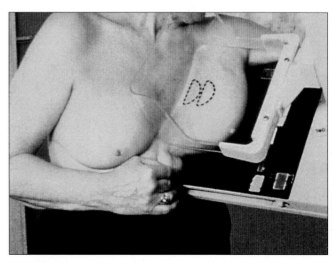

1.10 Patient undergoing mammography. The process can be uncomfortable.

Ultrasound (Figures 1.14, 1.15)

In ultrasound, high-frequency sound waves are passed through the breast, and reflections are detected and converted into images. Breast ultrasound is dependent on the skill of the operator and the quality of the equipment but is safe, painless, and suitable for use in all ages. It is an extremely valuable method for investigation of specific areas of the breast, although not an ideal tool for screening the entire breast. It is recommended in all patients with a palpable or mammographic abnormality. In those with cancer, it is useful to guide core biopsy and assess size, multifocality, and the presence of lymph node metastases.

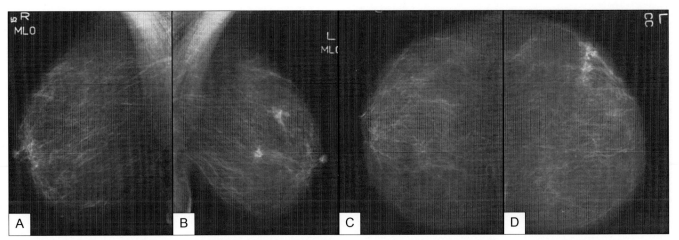

1.11A–D Normal arrangement of four mammograms viewed back to back. The pectoral muscle is seen in the upper corner of the mediolateral oblique (MLO) view (**A, B**). The label on the craniocaudal (CC) views is lateral (**C, D**). The mammograms show two small irregular opacities in the left breast due to multifocal breast cancer.

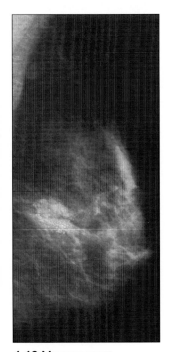

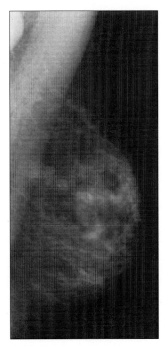

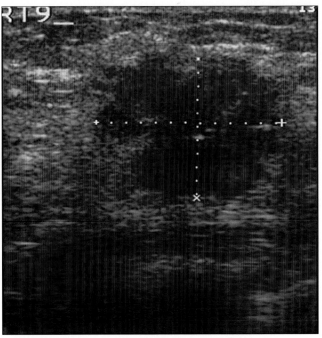

1.12 Mammogram showing a suspicious localized area of very heterogeneous calcification due to invasive breast cancer.

1.13 Mammogram showing an opacity high in the left axilla due to metastatic involvement of a lymph node from an occult breast primary.

1.14 Ultrasound scan image of a breast cancer. An irregular hypoechoic lesion typical of a cancer is visible. Cancers also often demonstrate posterior shadowing.

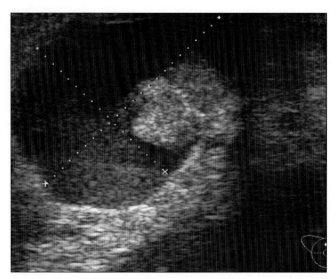

1.15 Ultrasound scan image showing a well-defined, anechoic lesion with posterior enhancement characteristic of a cyst but with a lesion visible on the back wall suspicious of an intracystic neoplasm. Aspiration of the cyst yielded bloodstained fluid and the lump did not disappear completely, raising clinical suspicions. The cyst quickly refilled. Histology revealed an encysted papillary carcinoma. These lesions are generally noninvasive and so nodal surgery is not required.

Magnetic resonance imaging (Figures 1.16, 1.17)

Magnetic resonance imaging (MRI) uses powerful magnets to affect the behaviour of hydrogen atoms and imaging software which allows the production of images. The equipment is expensive and specialist apparatus is required for breast imaging. The process can be noisy and claustrophobic for the patient. Particular expertise is required in the interpretation of images, and the exact role of MRI in breast investigation is still not clear (*Table 1.4*). It appears to be a sensitive technique for detecting invasive malignant breast lesions, but is not as sensitive for noninvasive disease. Its specificity is poor and it can result in an increase in potentially unnecessary further investigation, biopsy, resectional surgery (including mastectomy), and patient anxiety.

Table 1.4 Potential indications for breast MRI

- Screening in young, high-risk women (known or likely gene carriers)
- Investigation of suspicious areas in a previously operated breast
- Determination of size of known malignant lesion
- Investigation of occult breast primary with axillary metastasis
- Assessment of efficacy of neoadjuvant therapy
- Imaging of the breast in the presence of implants

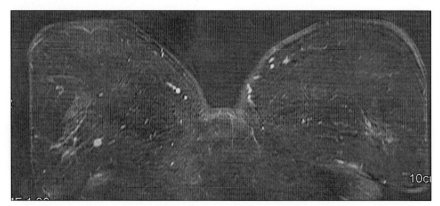

1.16 MRI scan of breasts with gadolinium enhancement, showing a small enhancing lesion on the right side due to a clinically and mammographically occult breast cancer in a woman who presented with axillary lymph node metastases. Time curves of uptake of contrast can also be useful in characterizing lesions.

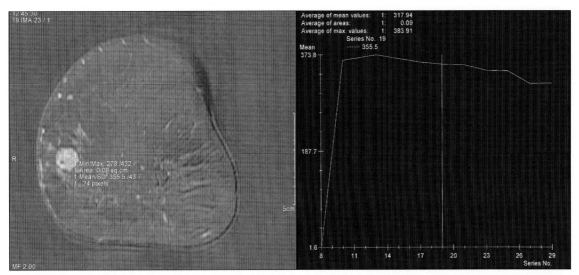

1.17 Contrast-enhanced MRI scan of the breast showing a similar enhancing lesion. The curve of the uptake of contrast in the lesion shows a rapid rise and then a slow decline. This is typically seen in malignant lesions and a cancer was confirmed on biopsy.

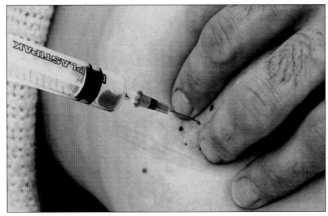

1.18 FNA of a solid breast lump. Suction is applied while the needle is moved in and out through the lesion. Usually less material is drawn up than is shown in the photograph. The aspirated material is spread on slides for cytological examination.

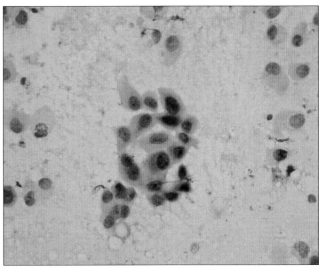

1.19 Cytology from FNA of confirmed carcinoma. Clustered and individual severely pleomorphic malignant epithelial cells. PAP stain, original magnification x20.

Pathological assessment

Fine needle aspiration cytology (Figures 1.18, 1.19)

Fine needle aspiration cytology involves the use of a 21- or 23-gauge needle and syringe to obtain cells from an area of concern within the breast or other structure. The cells are spread onto a microscope slide and prepared according to the preference of the pathologist. The procedure is quick but can be painful and a result can be obtained in less than 45 minutes.

Expertise on the part of the sampler and pathologist is necessary for reliable results, and the technique cannot differentiate between invasive and *in situ* malignancy. Definitive histology from core biopsy is recommended prior to axillary surgery, mastectomy, or neoadjuvant chemotherapy.

Core/vacuum-assisted biopsy (Figures 1.20–1.23)

A 14-gauge spring-loaded core needle biopsy can be performed with ease under local anaesthetic in the outpatient setting. Multiple cores are taken from the area of concern.

Vacuum assisted biopsy devices with larger bore needles are available allowing multiple cores to be taken without removal of the needle. These techniques provide the pathologist with more material to examine and a histological context and, therefore, may distinguish between invasive and noninvasive

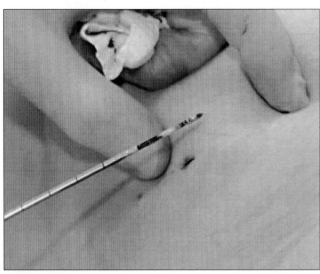

1.20 Needle core biopsy of a breast lesion. The biopsy is performed under local anaesthetic through a tiny stab incision. Multiple samples are usually taken. The process takes 10–15 minutes and can easily be performed in the outpatient clinic.

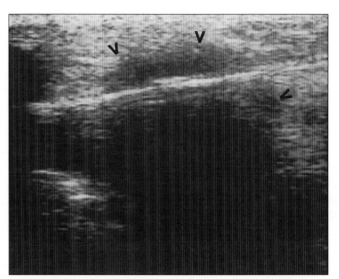

1.21 Ultrasound scan used to guide core biopsy and confirm sampling of the appropriate area. The image shows the bright white line of the needle passing through a poorly defined hypoechoic lesion due to a cancer (margin of the lesion is marked with arrows). Image guidance is increasingly used to ensure the appropriate area is sampled.

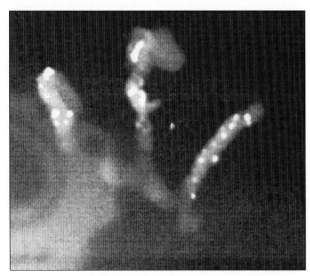

1.22 When core biopsy is performed for calcification within a breast it is important to confirm adequate calcifications have been sampled. This X-ray of core biopsies from an area of microcalcification confirms an adequate yield of calcifications.

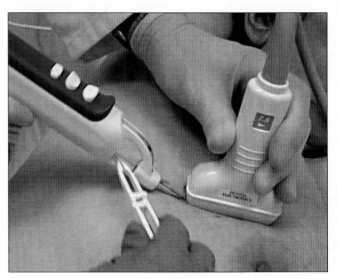

1.23 Vacuum assisted biopsy in progress. The procedure is performed under local anaesthetic. In contrast to the traditional core biopsy technique, the needle remains in place while multiple cores are taken. As in this case, ultrasound scanning is often used to guide the process.

malignancy and allow more accurate assessment of tumour type, grade, and hormone receptor status. Core biopsy can be performed in 10–15 minutes including the subsequent application of pressure to the sampled area to reduce bruising. Fixation and specimen preparation mean that histology is not available for 24–48 hours, although rapid processing procedures may mean that results can be available more quickly.

Ultrasound and radiological guidance are being used increasingly by both surgeons and radiologists to direct biopsy to ensure the appropriate area is sampled and to increase accuracy of diagnosis. Open surgical biopsy is seldom necessary and attempts should always be made to achieve a definitive diagnosis using needle biopsy techniques prior to such an operation.

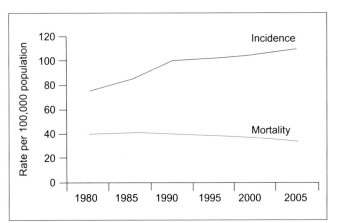

1.24 Changes in breast cancer incidence and mortality in the UK over time. Breast cancer incidence continues to increase while mortality is slowly falling.

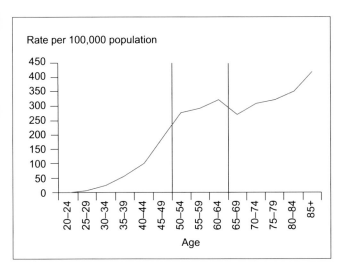

1.25 Change in incidence of breast cancer with age. There is a peak in cancer detection between 50 and 65 years due to screening.

EPIDEMIOLOGY OF BREAST CANCER

Epidemiology (Figures 1.24, 1.25)

Breast cancer is the commonest cancer in women, accounting for 15% of all cancers and 30% of cancers in women. In the UK, 48,034 breast cancers were diagnosed in 2008, 341 of these (0.7%) were in men. There were 12,116 deaths due to breast cancer in the UK in 2008 (accounting for 8% of all cancer deaths). Women currently have a 1 in 9 lifetime risk of developing breast cancer. The incidence of breast cancer increased by 13% between 1999 and 2008 although mortality is falling. Factors such as the ageing population, later first pregnancy, smaller family size, and the introduction of screening have made some contribution to the increasing incidence. The change in the organization of breast cancer management, with surgery being performed by breast specialists, more rational, widespread, and effective adjuvant treatment, and breast screening have contributed to the improvement in mortality.

Breast cancer incidence increases with age, oestrogen exposure, higher socioeconomic status, significant radiation exposure, family history, and specific predisposing conditions outlined above. The association with oestrogen exposure is reflected in an increased risk of breast cancer with early menarche, late menopause, reduced parity, postmenopausal obesity, and use of hormone replacement therapy (HRT). There is a weak association with oral contraceptive use and alcohol intake. Many of these factors are not amenable to intervention and are interrelated. An individual considering the use of HRT must weigh up the impact of menopausal symptoms on quality of life against the potential increased risk of breast cancer. HRT use effectively delays menopause and increases breast density, reducing the sensitivity of mammography, and delays the resolution of benign conditions such as breast cysts. There are substantial worldwide geographical variations in the incidence of breast cancer with the highest incidence in western Europe and North America. Oestrogen suppression reduces the incidence of breast cancer, but side-effects (including death) have meant that its use even in high-risk women in the general population is not currently recommended outside specific prevention trials.

Table 1.5 Potential strategy for classification and management of women at risk of familial breast cancer

Population risk
- Risk of developing breast cancer of <3% between ages 40 and 50 years and lifetime risk of <17%
- Those not fulfilling criteria below

Management
- Provision of written information regarding level of risk, breast awareness, and lifestyle (HRT, oral contraceptive use, diet, alcohol, breast feeding, family size, and timing)

Moderate risk
- Risk of developing breast cancer of 3–8% between ages 40 and 50 years and lifetime risk of 17–30%

Example family histories
- One first degree relative diagnosed with breast cancer at younger than 40 years, or
- Two first degree or second degree relatives diagnosed with breast cancer at an average age of older than 50 years, or
- Three first degree or second degree relatives diagnosed with breast cancer at an average age of older than 60 years

Management
- As above, plus
- Discussion of implications and limitations of early screening
- Option of audited annual mammography from age 40–49 to standards of NHS Breast Screening Programme

High risk
- Risk of developing breast cancer of >8% between ages 40 and 50 years and lifetime risk of >30%

Example family histories
At least the following female breast cancers only in the family:
- Two first degree or second degree relatives diagnosed with breast cancer at an average age of younger than 50 years (at least one of these must be a first degree relative), or
- Three first degree or second degree relatives diagnosed with breast cancer at an average age of younger than 60 years (at least one of these must be a first degree relative), or

- Four relatives diagnosed with breast cancer at any age (at least one of these must be a first degree relative)

Or
Families containing one relative with ovarian cancer at any age and, on the same side of the family:
- One first degree relative (including the relative with ovarian cancer) or second degree relative diagnosed with breast cancer at younger than 50 years, or
- Two first degree or second degree relatives diagnosed with breast cancer at an average age of younger than 60 years, or
- Another ovarian cancer at any age

Or
Families containing bilateral cancer (each breast cancer has the same count value as one relative):
- One first degree relative with cancer diagnosed in both breasts at an average age of younger than 50 years, or
- One first degree or second degree relative diagnosed with bilateral breast cancer and one first degree or second degree relative diagnosed with breast cancer at an average age of younger than 60 years

Or
Families containing male breast cancer at any age and on the same side of the family, and at least:
- One first degree or second degree relative diagnosed with breast cancer at younger than 50 years, or
- Two first degree or second degree relatives diagnosed with breast cancer at an average age of younger than 60 years

Management
- As above, plus
- Genetic counselling
- Consideration of genetic testing (if appropriate)
- Discussion of risk-reducing surgery

For those at highest risk, including those with known genetic mutation, annual screening with MRI is now recommended

(Adapted from: Familial Breast Cancer. *NICE Clinical Guideline 41*, October 2006)

Genetics (Figure 1.26)

The majority of breast cancers occur without any obvious genetic predisposition. Approximately 5% of breast cancers do appear to occur due to an inherited genetic abnormality in an autosomal dominant manner with incomplete penetrance. Two genes which predispose to breast cancer were identified in the mid-1990s – BRCA1 on chromosome 17 and BRCA2 on chromosome 13. Both are large genes with functions related to DNA repair and various mutations result in malignancy. Molecular screening for abnormalities in individuals at risk can be cumbersome and the situation has been complicated by the fact that both genes were patented.

A mutation of BRCA1 gene confers a lifetime risk of breast cancer of around 75% in addition to an increased risk of ovarian, prostate, and colon cancer. Disease onset is typically at a relatively early age. Mutation of the BRCA2 gene results in a lifetime risk of breast cancer of around 60%, again with disease onset at a relatively early age. Risk of ovarian cancer is increased and cases of male breast cancer are common. Mutations of p53 and PTEN genes are rare and predispose not only to breast cancer but to other cancers in affected families.

The majority of individuals thought on the basis of their family history to have a genetically inherited breast cancer will not be found to have mutation of a known predisposing gene, and it is likely that other genes remain to be recognized. It is over 10 years since the BRCA1 and 2 genes were identified, and any further predisposing genes are likely to give rise to small numbers of cases or have a low penetrance.

In those with an inherited mutation of a gene predisposing to breast cancer, the risk of death from breast cancer can be reduced by prophylactic mastectomy. Oestrogen suppression, oophorectomy or oestrogen receptor antagonism also reduces the incidence of breast cancer in this group.

Breast units should have a policy for management of those with a family history of breast cancer (*Table 1.5*). Having one or more relatives with breast cancer is not unusual and concerned individuals should be ranked into low, medium, or high-risk groups on the basis of their family history. Those at medium or high risk, who will often have several affected close relatives or relatives diagnosed at a young age, are offered early mammography and clinical examination although these have not been shown to affect outcome in this group. The role of MRI for screening is being assessed and it is now recommended for those at highest risk. Genetic analysis may be offered to those at high risk after appropriate counselling. Prophylactic mastectomy or oophorectomy should be discussed with gene carriers with full psychological support.

BREAST SCREENING

Screening (Figures 1.27–1.29)

Screening is the assessment of asymptomatic individuals in an effort to detect a serious condition at an early stage for which early intervention is beneficial.

Breast screening was introduced in the UK in 1988 following the recommendations of the Forrest Report, based on a review of the available evidence at the time. Quality

1.26 The pedigree of a family with a BRCA1 mutation. Known gene carriers are shown by filled symbols. All offspring of a gene carrier have a 50% chance of inheriting the mutation.

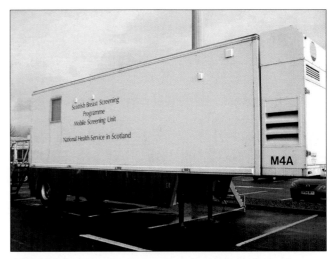

1.27 Mobile breast cancer screening unit deployed in a supermarket car park for the convenience of those attending for screening mammograms.

assurance was introduced as part of the screening process which has had beneficial effects on the evolution of symptomatic breast practice and beyond. Women are invited for mammography every 3 years between the ages of 50 and 70 years. Two views of each breast are taken at the first visit with reading of films by two radiologists. If the film is unsatisfactory or abnormal, the patient is recalled for further assessment in the screening service and further imaging and/or biopsy is performed. The screening service in England is under review and a change in the age range is planned.

Breast screening has been reported to save 1400 lives per year at a cost of £30,000 per year of life saved in the UK. For every 400 women screened over a 10-year period, it is calculated that one fewer women dies from breast cancer than would have died had they not been screened. This equates to 1 in 8 fewer breast cancer deaths in the target age group. The overall impact of breast screening remains contentious. Approximately 1 in 8 women with cancer diagnosed by screening would never have had their cancer diagnosed if they had not undergone screening. Over a 10-year period, 1 in 8 of all women screened will be recalled at least once. The breast screening process has changed the pattern of breast cancers seen with many more small, low-grade cancers and preinvasive lesions now being diagnosed and treated.

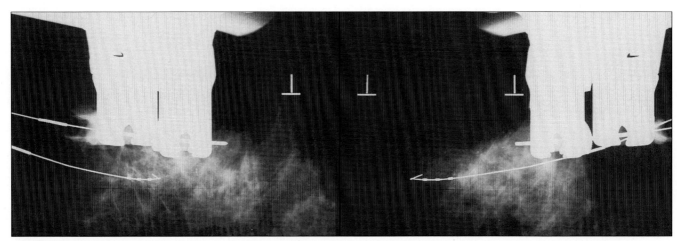

1.28 Radiological placement of wires to guide surgical excision. An area of microcalcification has been found on screening mammography and stereo biopsy has confirmed ductal carcinoma *in situ*. To guide excision, two wires are being placed to bracket the abnormality. Stereo images are taken 30° apart to confirm wire placement in the correct position in three dimensions. Stereo biopsy is performed in a similar manner.

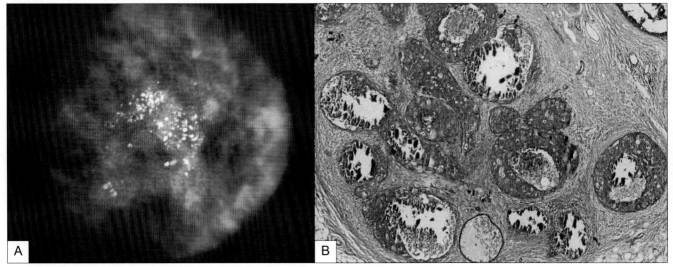

1.29A, B Specimen X-ray following excision of an area of coarse microcalcification identified at breast screening (**A**), with paired section showing high-grade DCIS with comedo necrosis and luminal calcification (**B**).

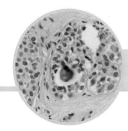
Histology and Staging

NONINVASIVE MALIGNANCIES AND CONDITIONS OF UNCERTAIN MALIGNANT POTENTIAL

Noninvasive malignancies (Figures 2.1–2.5)

A variety of abnormalities can be identified in the cells lining the terminal duct lobular units short of an invasive malignant appearance penetrating the basement membrane. These include usual type hyperplasia, atypical hyperplasia, and noninvasive (*in situ*) carcinoma. Ductal and lobular patterns of atypical hyperplasia and *in situ* cancer can be recognized from the histological pattern of disease and cell type. Ductal carcinoma *in situ* is the most common form of noninvasive carcinoma (making up 4% of symptomatic and 25% of screen-detected 'cancers'). It is characterized by distortion, distention, and complete involvement by a homogenous and neoplastic population of cells in adjacent ducts and lobular units. By contrast, lobular carcinoma *in situ* is rare (<1% of

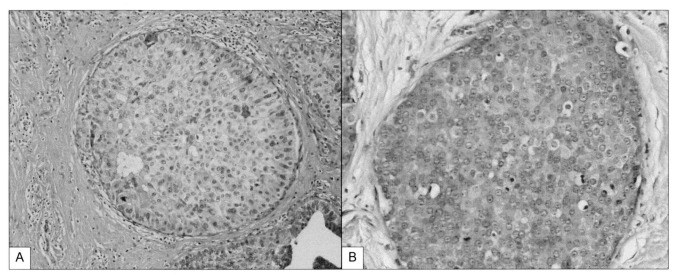

2.1 Photomicrograph on left (**A**) shows a duct space filled with a mixture of atypical epithelial cells with admixed myoepithelial cells. The lesion does not meet the criteria for a diagnosis of DCIS and the designation 'ADH' is appropriate. Photomicrograph on right (**B**) shows a duct space replaced by a pure population of malignant ductal epithelial cells (DCIS) of intermediate grade.

screen-detected 'cancers') and exhibits relatively uniform expansion of the whole lobule by regular cells with regular, round or oval nuclei. While each involved lobular unit has a uniform cellular population, the pattern and even cytology may, and often does, vary between units with some intervening units being minimally involved or uninvolved. Some patients present with combined features that should be regarded as having clinical features of both processes.

Criteria have been agreed to distinguish atypical ductal hyperplasia (ADH) from ductal carcinoma *in situ* (DCIS). Difficulty in distinguishing atypical lobular hyperplasia (ALH) and lobular carcinoma *in situ* (LCIS) has led to them often being grouped together as lobular *in situ* neoplasia (LIN). In general, lesions that involve only a few membrane bound spaces and that measure less than 2–4 mm in their greatest diameter should be regarded as hyperplastic lesions (with or without atypia) and not *in situ* carcinoma (*Table 2.1*). Whether there is progression over time of hyperplasia to *in situ* disease to invasive carcinoma with increasing genetic mutations within the affected cells analogous to the adenoma/carcinoma sequence of colorectal neoplasia, is not entirely clear.

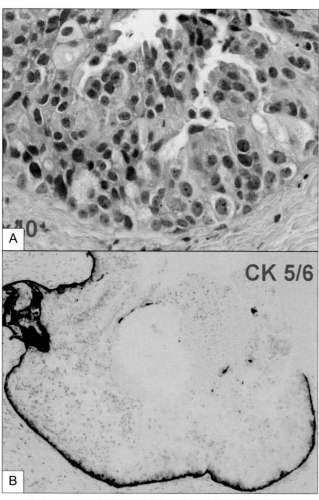

2.2 High-grade DCIS (**A**), The CK 5/6 stain (**B**) picks out the intact myoepithelial layer around the periphery of the duct, while the *in situ* carcinoma cells that fill the duct show no staining. This stain helps to confirm that the tumour is not invasive.

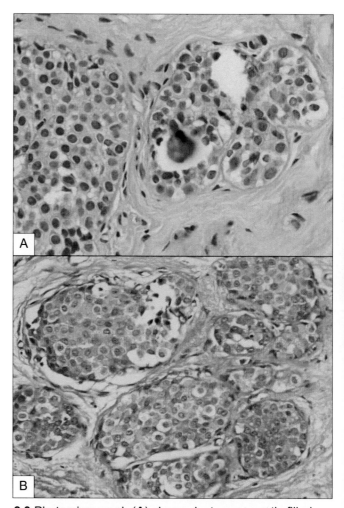

2.3 Photomicrograph (**A**) shows duct space partly filled with a population of lobular epithelial cells – ALH. Associated microcalcification is common in these lesions. Photomicrograph (**B**) shows a similar pattern, but the lobules are now completely filled and expanded by atypical lobular epithelial cells – LCIS. It is recognized that the distinction between ALH and LCIS is not easy and a preferred blanket term for the proliferation is '*in situ* lobular neoplasia'.

Table 2.1 Classification of ductal carcinoma *in situ*

By grade	By architectural pattern
Low	Cribriform
Intermediate	Solid
High	Flat or clinging
	Micropapillary
	Papillary
	Apocrine

Notes:

1 Grade is determined by nuclear features only

2 There is no consistent relationship between grade and pattern with the exception of cribriform DCIS which is usually low or intermediate grade

3 Micropapillary DCIS is frequently multifocal

4 Comedo necrosis is most commonly seen in high grade lesions

Those with atypical hyperplasia and carcinoma *in situ* are at increased risk of invasive disease, but the timescale is measured in years and it may not occur at all in many individuals. Development of invasive carcinoma can also occur at some distance from the noninvasive disease. Different histological characteristics of *in situ* disease are recognized which correspond with subsequent risk of progression and recurrence.

Approximately 40% of those with low-grade ductal carcinoma *in situ* will develop invasive cancer over a 30-year period, with the majority of these developing within the first decade. About 15–20% of women with a diagnosis of lobular carcinoma *in situ* will develop breast cancer in the same breast, and a further 10–15% will develop an invasive carcinoma in the contralateral breast.

Atypical hyperplasia and carcinoma *in situ* are usually asymptomatic, although a lump is palpable in a small proportion of those with DCIS, and Paget's disease is often seen in association with DCIS.

It is recommended that if atypical hyperplasia or LIN is diagnosed on core biopsy, then formal excision of the area should be performed as these conditions can be associated with adjacent invasive cancer. In general, once a diagnostic

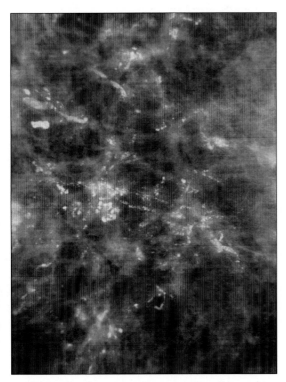

2.4 Magnification view mammogram of an area of suspicious microcalcification due to ductal carcinoma *in situ*.

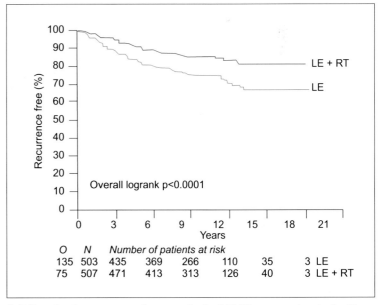

2.5 Graph of recurrence-free survival of 1010 women treated with or without radiotherapy to the breast, following wide excision of ductal carcinoma *in situ* (with no disease at margins) in the EORTC 10853 trial. Risk of recurrence is almost halved by radiotherapy (hazard ratio 0.53, p<0.0001) but the absolute benefit may be small, particularly for some groups. O, observed number of events; N, number of patients; LE, local excision; RT, radiotherapy. (Adapted from Bijker N, *et al.* [2006]. *J Clin Oncol* **24**:3381–87.)

biopsy has shown atypical hyperplasia or LIN no further surgical treatment is necessary, but long-term review with annual mammography is recommended. Clear margins are not necessary and these abnormalities appear to be a marker of general risk. Anti-oestrogen therapy with tamoxifen or raloxifene reduces the risk of subsequent invasive cancer in atypical hyperplasia and LIN, although the proportion of patients who benefit is small.

DCIS requires wide excision to clear margins as the risk of progression to invasive cancer is substantial, particularly for intermediate and high-grade DCIS; if excision is incomplete, recurrence is at a rate of at least 2% per annum. When recurrence occurs after excision, the disease is invasive in 50% of cases. Adjuvant radiotherapy to the affected breast and anti-oestrogen therapy reduce the risk of recurrence, and their use depends on hormone receptor status and the risk of recurrence in each case. Long-term review with annual mammography is recommended (*Table 2.2*).

Paget's disease (Figures 2.6, 2.7)

Paget's disease of the nipple arises when malignant cells spread to involve the epithelium of the nipple skin resulting in a red, scaling appearance which can sometimes be difficult to differentiate from eczema. Paget's disease always involves the nipple and may spread beyond the nipple to involve the surrounding areolar area, whereas eczema starts on the areola and usually spares the nipple. If there is concern that Paget's disease is present, a punch biopsy or a core biopsy including nipple skin should be performed under local anaesthetic in the outpatient clinic. If Paget's disease is confirmed, further investigation is required to determine whether an underlying invasive malignancy is present.

Table 2.2 Suggested management of lobular *in situ* neoplasia, atypical ductal hyperplasia, or ductal carcinoma *in situ* on biopsy

Biopsy result	Surgery	Further management
Lobular *in situ* neoplasia or ADH	Excision biopsy to ensure invasive disease/DCIS not missed	Observation with annual mammography Consider endocrine therapy
Ductal carcinoma *in situ*	Wide excision to clear margins (may require mastectomy)	Consider radiotherapy (unless mastectomy) or endocrine therapy/trial enrolment Observation with annual mammography

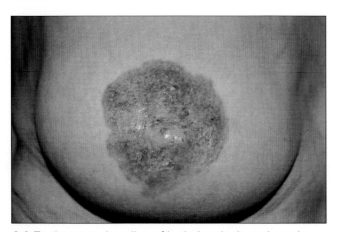

2.6 Erythema and scaling of both the nipple and areola due to Paget's disease of the nipple.

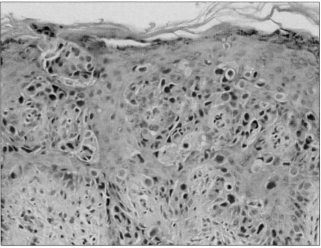

2.7 Paget's disease of the nipple. Epidermis of the nipple is infiltrated by nests of malignant cells. H&E, original magnification x4.

HISTOLOGY OF BREAST CANCER

Histological types (Figures 2.8–2.10)

The vast majority of breast cancers arise from epithelial cells lining the terminal duct lobular unit. Some tumours do show distinct patterns of growth and cellular morphology, and on this basis certain types of breast cancer can be identified. Those with specific features are called invasive carcinomas of special type, while the remainder are considered to be of no special type. This classification has clinical relevance in that certain special type tumours have a much better prognosis than tumours that are of no special type.

Approximately 80% of breast cancers are of no special type. Lobular cancers account for around 10% of all invasive cancers. These are often more difficult to diagnose and their

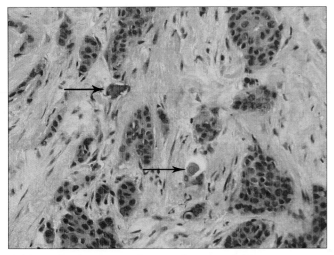

2.8 Invasive breast carcinoma of no special type. Infiltrating nests of carcinoma cells. Note two small stromal microcalcifications (arrows). These are often detected on mammograms.

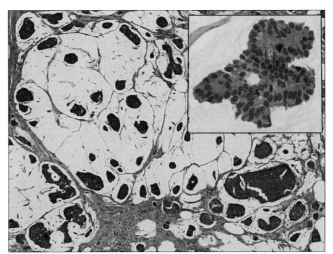

2.9 Invasive mucinous carcinoma. One of the 'special types' of carcinoma. Note islands of tumour cells set in a background of mucoid material which stains a pale bluish-pink with H&E. These tumours have a better prognosis than no special type and lobular carcinomas. H&E, original magnification x10 and x40 (insert).

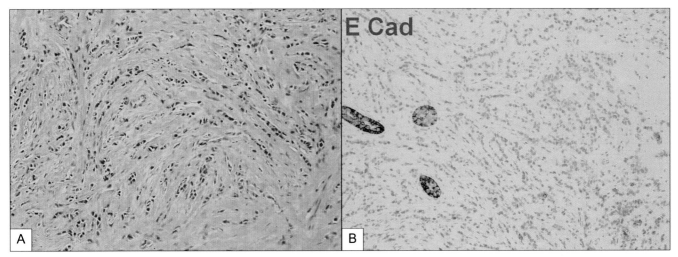

2.10 Invasive lobular carcinoma. **A**: Note stromal infiltration by cords of small carcinoma cells showing a single file pattern. E-cadherin staining. **B**: A number of small normal ducts show strong positive staining of epithelial cells, while the invasive carcinoma cells are completely negative.

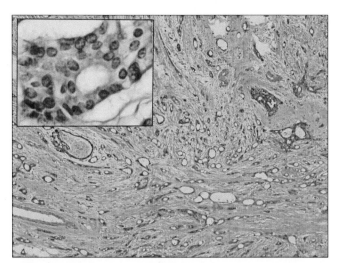

2.11 Invasive carcinoma NST Grade I. Note prominent tubule formation and small to intermediate sized nuclei with little pleomorphism (insert). H&E, original magnification x4 and x40 (insert).

size is often underestimated clinically, resulting in a higher rate of incomplete excision. Special types of breast cancer are less common and include tubular, cribriform, mucinous or mucoid, medullary, and papillary.

Grade (Figures 2.11–2.14)

Prognostic information can be gained by grading the degree of differentiation of the tumour. Degrees of glandular formation, nuclear pleomorphism, and frequency of mitoses are scored from 1 to 3. These values are combined and converted into three groups: grade I (score 3–5), grade II (scores 6 and 7), and grade III (scores 8 and 9). This derived histological grade (known as the Bloom and Richardson grade or the Scarff, Bloom, and Richardson grade) is an important predictor of both disease-free and overall survival.

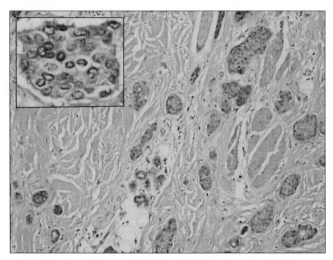

2.12 Invasive carcinoma NST Grade II. Predominantly solid nests of tumour with intermediate sized nuclei with only mild pleomorphism (insert). H&E, original magnification x4 and x40 (insert).

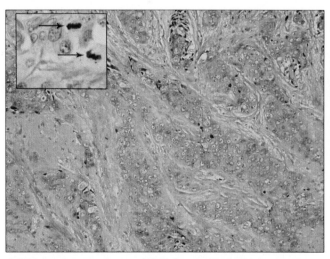

2.13 Invasive carcinoma NST Grade III. Solid nests of tumour cells showing nuclear pleomorphism and frequent mitoses (arrows on insert). H&E, original magnification x10 and x40 (insert).

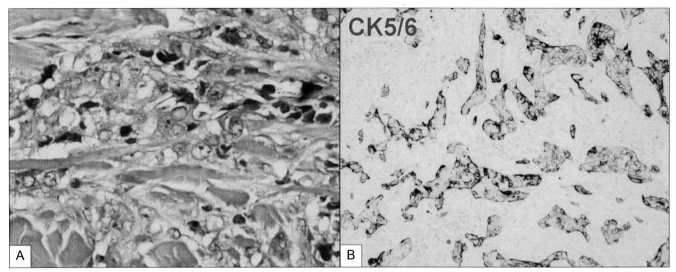

2.14 A: Grade III invasive carcinoma of basal phenotype. Approximately 20% of grade III carcinomas of the breast are of a basal phenotype and show positive staining with basal markers such as CK 5/6, P63, or smooth muscle actin. These tumours are usually ER, PGR, and HER 2 negative and are more aggressive than those of luminal phenotype (the usual type of breast cancer). **B**: Positive CK 5/6 staining of invasive tumour cells typical of basal phenotype.

Lymphovascular invasion (Figure 2.15)

The presence of cancer cells in blood or lymphatic vessels is a marker of more aggressive disease, and patients with this feature are at increased risk of both local and systemic recurrence.

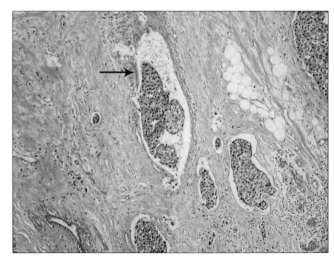

2.15 Venous (arrow) and lymphatic invasion by carcinoma of breast. H&E, original magnification x10.

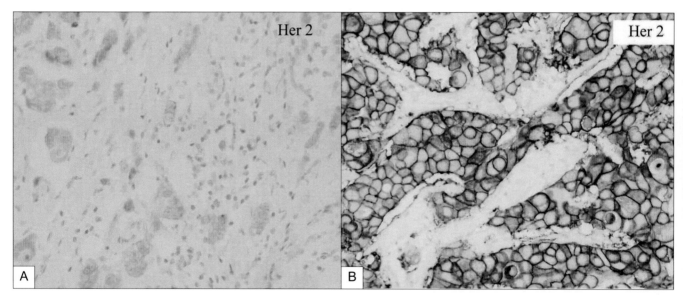

2.16 A: Grade III invasive carcinoma showing patchy low-intensity nuclear staining for oestrogen receptor (ER). The Allred score for this is 5 (proportion score 4; intensity score 1) (moderately positive). **B**: Invasive lobular carcinoma showing strongly positive nuclear staining for ER. The Allred score for this example is 8 (proportion score 5; intensity score 3) (maximum score).

2.17 A: Invasive carcinoma showing weak discontinuous membrane staining for HER2. This is an example of a negative test (score 1+). **B**: Invasive carcinoma showing strong continuous membrane staining for HER2. This is an example of a positive test (score 3+).

Hormone and growth factor receptors (Figures 2.16–2.19)

Approximately 75% of breast cancers bear receptors on their cells for oestrogen, activation of which stimulates cell growth. The proportion of cells bearing receptors and the number of receptors per cell may vary and is assessed by the Allred score. The greater the level of receptor the more likely the cancer is to respond to anti-oestrogen treatment.

The HER2 growth factor receptor is overexpressed on about 20% of breast cancers. HER2 has long been recognized as a marker of poor prognosis in breast cancer. Overexpression of HER2 predicts response to antiHER2 agents.

A subset of cancers (including basal cancers [2.14]) have no oestrogen, progesterone or HER2 receptors. These are referred to as triple negative and also have a poorer prognosis.

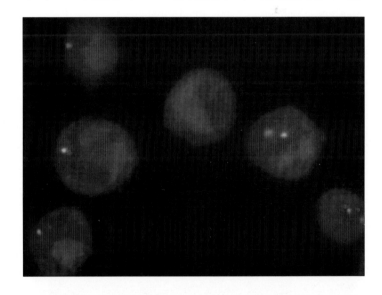

2.18 FISH testing for the HER2 gene located on chromosome 17 is regarded as the 'gold standard' for assessing gene amplification at the present time. Current guidelines recommend FISH testing of all equivocal cases (2+) identified by immunohistochemistry. In the illustrations shown, the red probe identifies copies of the HER2 gene (one dot per copy) while the green probe locates the centromere of chromosome 17. True gene amplification is shown by an increased ratio (above 2) of the HER2 gene copy number compared with the chromosome 17 number. In this example, the HER2 gene is **not** amplified, with a ratio of red dots to green dots approximating 1.

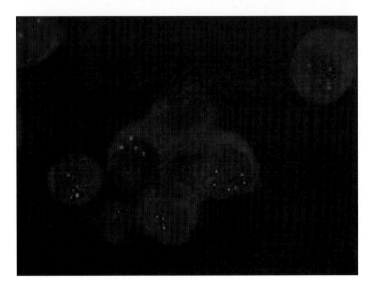

2.19 FISH for HER2 showing striking amplification of the HER2 gene with increased copy numbers marked by the red dots. In this example, the gene copy:chromosome 17 ratio is approximately 5.

STAGING OF BREAST CANCER

Staging classification (Figures 2.20–2.22)

When the diagnosis of a breast cancer has been made, the patient should be informed in a compassionate manner by an experienced clinician and introduced to a breast care nurse who acts as a point of future contact and provides information and support. To determine the most appropriate management plan it is important to know the stage or extent of disease. The UICC (Union Internationale Contre le Cancre) TNM (Tumour/Node/Metastasis) classification is commonly used but is not ideally suited to breast cancer (*Table 2.3*). Clinical examination provides some information of the likely size of the lesion, the presence of involvement of the skin or chest wall, and whether the cancer has inflammatory features. Clinical assessment of axillary and supraclavicular lymph node involvement is essential but insensitive. To improve the TNM system, a separate

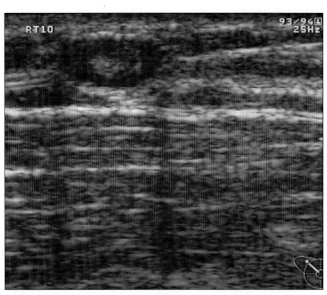

2.20 Ultrasound scan of a normal small intramammary lymph node in the axillary tail with hypoechoic cortex and bright central medulla.

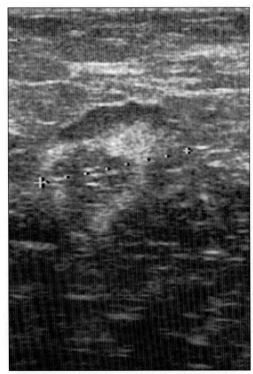

2.21 Enlarged lymph node in axilla with abnormal and irregular appearance due to metastatic involvement. Irregularities of the lymph node cortex or a cortical thickness of greater than 2 mm raise suspicions of metastasis.

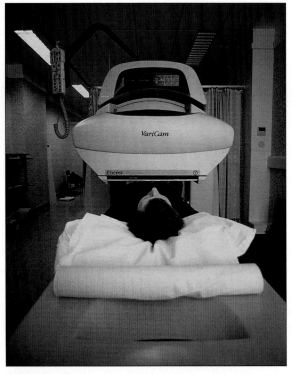

2.22 A bone scan in progress. About 4 hours after injection of 600 MBq technetium-labelled methylene diphosphonate, the patient is scanned. The label concentrates in active areas of bone and is used to attempt to exclude bone metastases as part of preoperative staging.

Table 2.3 TNM staging

T – Primary tumour

TX   Primary tumour cannot be assessed

T0   No evidence of primary tumour

Tis   Carcinoma *in situ*: intraductal carcinoma, or lobular carcinoma *in situ*, or Paget's disease of the nipple with no tumour

T1   Tumour 2 cm or less in greatest dimension

T1mic Microinvasion 0.1 cm or less in greatest dimension

T1a   More than 0.1 cm but not more than 0.5 cm in greatest dimension

T1b   More than 0.5 cm but not more than 1 cm in greatest dimension

T1c   More than 1 cm but not more than 2 cm in greatest dimension

T2   Tumour more than 2 cm but not more than 5 cm in greatest dimension

T3   Tumour more than 5 cm in greatest dimension

T4   Tumour of any size with direct extension to chest wall or skin

T4a   Extension to chest wall wall (not including pectoralis muscle)

T4b   Oedema (including *peau d'orange*), or ulceration of the skin of the breast, or satellite skin nodules confined to the same breast

T4c   Both 4a and 4b, above

T4d   Inflammatory carcinoma

N – Regional lymph nodes

NX   Regional lymph nodes cannot be assessed (e.g. previously removed)

N0   No regional lymph node metastasis

N1   Metastasis to movable ipsilateral axillary node(s)

N2   Metastasis to ipsilateral axillary node(s) fixed to one another or to other structures, or clinically apparent ipsilateral internal mammary nodes in absence of axillary node metastasis

N2a   Metastasis to ipsilateral axillary node(s) fixed to one another or to other structures

N2b   Metastasis only in clinically apparent internal mammary nodes in absence of clinically evident axillary node metastasis

N3   Metastasis to ipsilateral infraclavicular node(s), or ipsilateral internal mammary lymph node(s) with axillary lymph node metastasis, or metastasis in ipsilateral supraclavicular node(s)

N3a   Metastasis in ipsilateral infraclavicular node(s)

N3b   Metastasis in ipsilateral internal mammary lymph node(s) and axillary lymph node(s)

N3c   Metastasis in ipsilateral supraclavicular node(s)

M – Distant metastasis

MX   Distant metastasis cannot be assessed

M0   No distant metastasis

M1   Distant metastasis

Summary of stages:

Stage 0   Carcinoma *in situ*

Stage IA   T1 N0

Stage IB   T1 with nodal micrometastasis

Stage IIA   T2 N0 or T1N1

Stage IIB   T3 N0 or T2 N1

Stage IIIA   T1 or 2 N2 or T3 N1

Stage IIIB   T4 N0-2

Stage IIIC   Any T N3

Stage IV   Distant metastasis (M)

Notes

1 Paget's disease associated with a tumour is classified according to the size of the tumour.

2 Microinvasion is the extension of cancer cells beyond the basement membrane into the adjacent tissues with no focus more than 0.1 cm in greatest dimension. When there are multiple foci of microinvasion, the size of only the largest focus is used to classify the microinvasion. (Do not use the sum of all the individual foci.) The presence of multiple foci of microinvasion should be noted, as it is with multiple larger invasive carcinomas.

3 Chest wall includes ribs, intercostal muscles, and serratus anterior muscle but not pectoral muscle.

4 Inflammatory carcinoma of the breast is characterized by diffuse, brawny induration of the skin with an erysipeloid edge, usually with no underlying mass. If the skin biopsy is negative and there is no localized measurable primary cancer, the T category is pTX when pathologically staging a clinical inflammatory carcinoma (T4d). Dimpling of the skin, nipple retraction, or other skin changes, except those in T4b and T4d, may occur in T1, T2, or T3 without affecting the classification.

Source: International Union Against Cancer (UICC) (2009). *TNM Classification of Malignant Tumours*. LH Sobin, *et al.* (eds), 7th edn. Wiley-Blackwell, New York.

pathological classification has been added which allows tumour size and node status, as assessed by a pathologist, to be taken into account. Prognosis in breast cancer relates to the stage of the disease at presentation.

Systemic metastatic disease may be suspected from the history or on clinical examination. Mammography, ultrasound, and MRI scanning can all be used to estimate tumour size and detect multifocality, and imaging provides a more accurate assessment of tumour size than clinical measurement. Ultrasound scanning is being used increasingly to look for involved axillary lymph nodes at diagnosis. Metastatic disease is uncommon in women presenting with apparently early breast cancer and, therefore, a selective approach is usually taken to further investigations. Blood sampling for full blood count, urea, electrolytes, liver function tests, and calcium and perhaps a chest X-ray are recommended for the majority as these are also of value as part of a preoperative assessment. For patients at higher risk of metastatic disease such as those with larger tumours, obviously enlarged axillary lymph nodes, those with signs of local advancement, or symptoms or blood tests suggestive of metastases further investigation with liver ultrasound scanning, bone scanning, computed tomography (CT), MRI, or positron emission tomography (PET) scans may be valuable.

The aim of staging is to separate patients suitable for a radical, potentially curative combination of loco-regional treatments followed by appropriate adjuvant systemic therapy from those with metastatic disease, who are treated primarily with systemic therapy. Imaging of metastatic disease as part of staging also assists in appropriate and targeted treatment selection, and is useful for monitoring the effectiveness of therapy.

For ease of management, breast cancer can be classified into three separate groups based on disease extent: (1) early or operable breast cancer, (2) locally advanced disease, and (3) metastatic breast cancer.

Multidisciplinary team working (Figure 2.23)

The cornerstone of management of individuals with all cancers is multidisciplinary team working. The components of the multidisciplinary team will vary but may include specialist breast surgeons, radiologists, pathologists, clinical and medical oncologists, plastic surgeons, breast care nurses, research, and audit staff. The forum for team working will vary but is often based around a meeting held at least weekly. Teleconferencing is increasingly helping more peripheral units to have access to specialists who may not be based at their institution.

Any individual diagnosed with breast cancer should be discussed at diagnosis and when any further intervention is contemplated. It is also useful to discuss those with nonconcordant investigation findings. A written unit policy is useful and accurate record keeping is essential.

Psychological aspects

A diagnosis of breast cancer has a profound impact on the patient and their family. The patient may be undergoing treatment which can substantially affect body image and their general well-being. Patients also have numerous correct and incorrect preconceived ideas of what the diagnosis and treatment will involve. It is not surprising, therefore, that depression and anxiety are common, particularly in the first year of diagnosis, as are emotional, sexual, and financial problems. The team involved in managing patients with breast cancer must be sensitive to these problems and be in a position to provide appropriate support and referral for appropriate treatments if required.

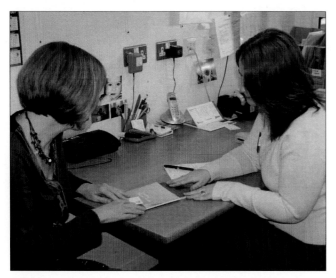

2.23 All patients diagnosed with breast cancer should meet with a specialist nurse experienced in the management of such patients to provide information, advice, and support.

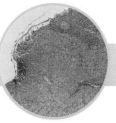

Chapter 3

Treatment of Breast Cancer

LOCAL TREATMENT OF EARLY BREAST CANCER

Treatment components (Figure 3.1)

There are three components of the treatment of breast cancer: (1) local treatment of the cancer in the breast, (2) treatment of the loco-regional draining nodes, principally in the axilla, and (3) systemic treatments to eradicate any disease which may be present outwith the breast and loco-regional nodal basins. Breast cancer is uncommon in men and may present at a more advanced stage because of a smaller volume of breast tissue; however, the principles of management are the same in women and men.

Early (operable) disease

Breast (Figures 3.2–3.7)
Initial treatment of the primary breast tumour in an individual with early or operable breast cancer is usually surgical. Some patients with locally advanced breast disease and most with

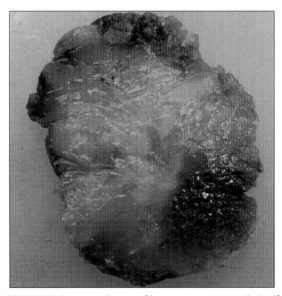

3.1 Mammograms of a male patient showing an irregular opacity on the left due to a breast cancer.

3.2 Wide excision specimen of breast cancer cut in half to show central tumour.

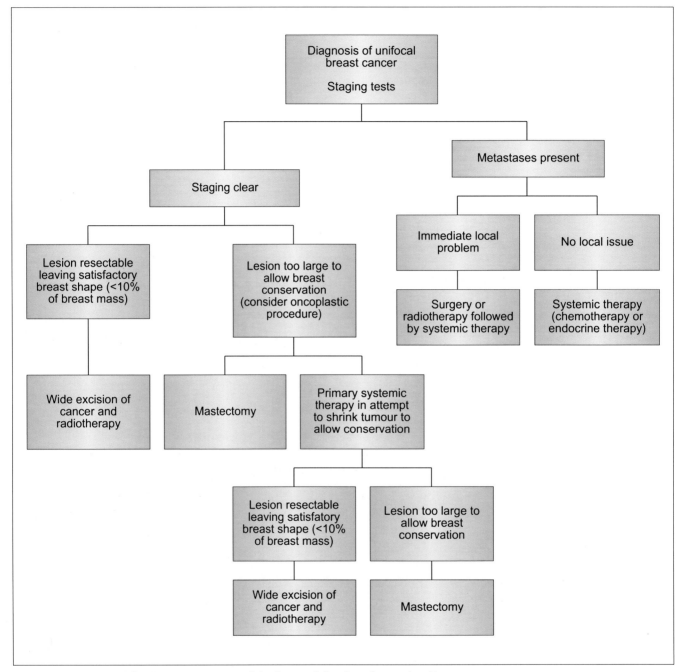

3.3 Potential protocol for the management of the breast following diagnosis of breast cancer.

cancers involving underlying muscle are suitable for a primary surgical approach, as long as other features such as inflammatory changes or distant metastatic disease are not present. The primary surgical options for management of the breast are mastectomy and breast conservation. Breast conservation therapy consists of excision of the tumour with a 1 cm macroscopic margin of normal tissue (wide local excision) plus breast radiotherapy. Controversy has surrounded how much extra tissue should be removed and what constitutes an involved or positive margin. Current evidence suggests that microscopic margins of 1 mm or more are adequate and that increasingly wide margins will not reduce local recurrence rates but will adversely affect cosmetic outcomes. Local recurrence rates should be less than 1% per annum following wide excision and radiotherapy.

There are lower levels of psychological morbidity with

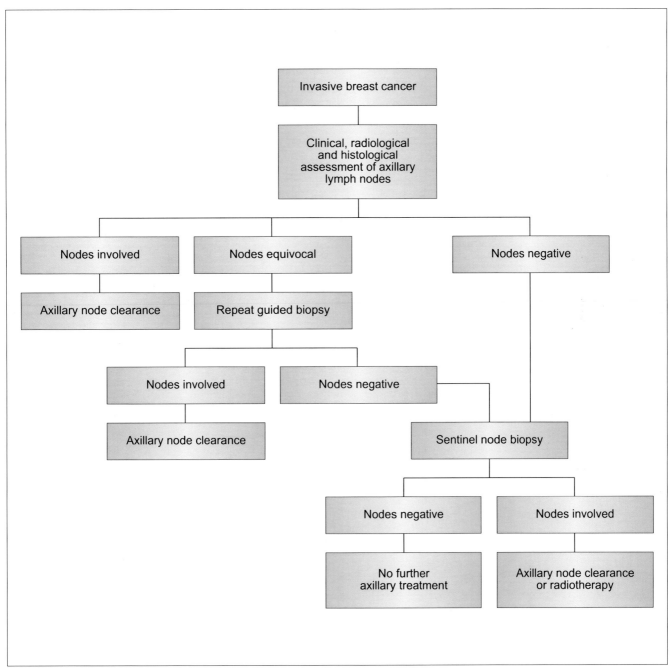

3.4 Potential protocol for management of the axilla following diagnosis of breast cancer.

breast conservation than with mastectomy; it also results in comparatively better body image, freedom of dress, sexuality, and self-esteem. More extensive excisions of a whole quadrant of the breast (quadrantectomy) have worse cosmetic outcomes and do not have a significantly lower local recurrence rate than wide excisions. There is no size limit for breast conservation surgery, but adequate excision of lesions over 4 cm generally produces a poor cosmetic result in all but women with very large breasts, unless both breasts are reduced or the defect in the breast is filled by oncoplastic techniques. There is no age limit for breast conservation. The approach will depend on the size of the tumour in relation to the size of the breast, multifocality, and patient choice. Reasonable arm mobility is required to receive breast radiotherapy and if arm mobility is limited breast conservation may not be advisable.

Mastectomy (Figure 3.8)

Mastectomy involves removal of as much of the breast tissue on the affected side as possible. It is usually performed if the extent of disease is large in relation to the size of the breast, where there is proven multicentric disease, or where a patient prefers mastectomy. Patients sometimes choose mastectomy for disease suitable for breast conserving surgery because they think mastectomy has a better long-term survival. This is not true and once informed of this many are happy to choose breast conserving surgery.

Mastectomy is usually performed through a low transverse scar to leave a flat wound with no excess skin to allow easy placement of an external prosthesis. The nipple is usually removed with an ellipse of skin usually incorporating the skin directly over the cancer. It is important to plan incisions to avoid unsightly 'dog ears' at the medial and lateral ends of mastectomy wounds. Other options to help avoid this include using a breast reduction-type skin incision (Wise pattern) or 'fish tailing' the ends of the wounds. Skin flaps are raised in the plane between the breast and subcutaneous fat down to the chest wall and the breast is then dissected off the chest wall posteriorly, leaving the fascia overlying the pectoral muscle (unless there is invasion of underlying muscle, when sufficient muscle should be excised to completely remove the cancer). Mastectomy flaps can be sutured to the chest wall by a quilting technique which

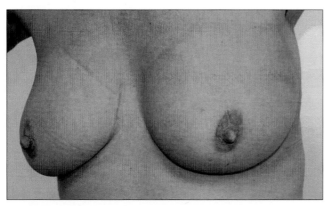

3.5 Well healed scar following breast conservation therapy with wide excision of the breast cancer and radiotherapy.

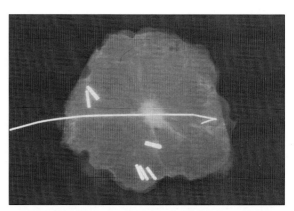

3.6 Specimen X-ray showing satisfactory margins following excision of a screen-detected, impalpable breast cancer. The lesion has been localized using a hooked wire and the specimen has been orientated using clips.

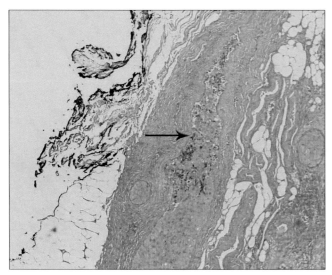

3.7 DCIS (arrow) extending close to the inked margin in a wide local excision specimen. H&E, original magnification x4.

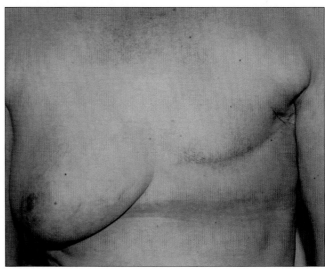

3.8 Scar following mastectomy and radiotherapy to the chest wall.

appears to reduce the rate of subsequent seroma. The wound should be closed with an absorbable subcuticular stitch. If reconstruction is being undertaken, more skin (including the nipple in some circumstances) may be preserved (skin-sparing mastectomy). Drains are often placed following surgery and these are left until drainage is below a threshold volume, or are routinely removed after a few days depending on local protocol. Complications include bleeding, infection, and necrosis of the wound edge. Some degree of numbness of the skin flaps is expected and seroma formation is common.

Breast conservation

If a unifocal breast cancer can be completely excised with a satisfactory margin without significantly deforming the breast, wide excision of the cancer should be considered. In general, around 10% of the breast volume can be excised without deformity although this proportion may be less for tumours in the medial part of the breast. It is not necessary to remove skin over the cancer. The nipple may be excised with the cancer if it lies in close relation or if malignant nipple discharge is present. The skin envelope and tissue within the breast can be mobilized to minimize any defect produced by wide excision.

The increasing recognition of impalpable cancers (and noninvasive disease) has led to an increase in the need for collaboration with radiology in aiding excision of these lesions. One or more hooked wires can be placed through the lesions guided by ultrasound scanning or stereo radiography. The wires are then used as a guide to excision by the surgeon. Guided injection of radiolabel around the lesion and intraoperative use of a hand-held, gamma radiation-detection probe to guide surgery can also be used. Orientation of the specimen aids pathological assessment and X-ray of the excision specimen assists intraoperative assessment of complete removal of the lesion. If a breast cancer is thought to be too large to allow breast conservation at diagnosis, consideration may be given to primary treatment with endocrine or chemotherapy in an attempt to shrink the tumour and allow conservation.

Drains are not required after wide excision. Incomplete excision rates should be in the range of 10 to 25%. If there is disease at only a limited number of margins, re-excision of these margins can be performed at a second operation. If there is extensive margin involvement, mastectomy may be necessary. Other problems after breast conserving surgery are bleeding, infection, and poor cosmesis. Lymphoedema of the breast is also sometimes seen. Wide excision of breast cancer alone without postoperative radiotherapy has an unacceptable recurrence rate of around 30% and therefore wide excision should be followed by radiotherapy to the breast. Ongoing trials are assessing whether there is a group of older women or those with good-prognosis cancers who can safely avoid radiotherapy.

An aesthetic approach (Figure 3.9)

The aesthetic impact of all surgical interventions on the breast should be considered prior to the procedure, whether a needle biopsy or mastectomy. Incision placement should allow adequate access and the incision should be placed with consideration of the skin crease lines and how obtrusive the scar may be. Resection of skin or large amounts of breast tissue distorts the breast, particularly if followed by radiotherapy, and the effect of this should be considered. While a mastectomy always has a profound impact on body image, a flat scar without a dog ear of tissue at either end is crucial to allow placement of an external prosthesis and psychological adjustment to the procedure. Incision planning and the use of techniques to avoid unsightly wounds such as fishtailing may assist this.

The increasing awareness of oncoplastic techniques has allowed excision of large amounts of breast tissue without distorting the breast shape. This is performed by volume displacement – mobilization of breast tissue to minimize a

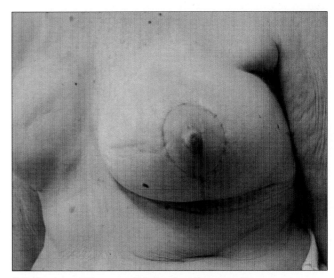

3.9 Postoperative result following therapeutic mammoplasty for large breast cancer. A good breast shape can be maintained with acceptable scarring. A large breast cancer has been excised and the breast reshaped as in a breast reduction procedure. The operative procedure takes longer and surgery on the normal contralateral breast is required. The blue staining on the skin in this case is from the patent blue dye used for sentinel node biopsy.

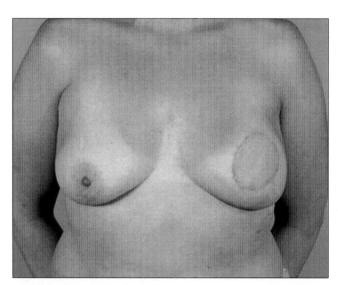

3.10 Left latissimus dorsi flap reconstruction. This patient has undergone a left mastectomy and axillary clearance with immediate reconstruction for a large central breast cancer. The breast has been reconstructed using a latissimus dorsi myocutaneous flap with an underlying breast implant.

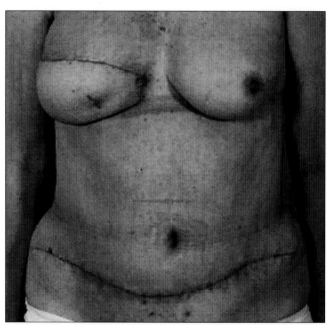

3.11 Following breast reconstruction using a free flap of lower abdominal tissue, the reconstructed right breast and abdominal scar are shown. The umbilicus is also brought through a hole in the abdominal skin to allow it to lie in a more natural position.

defect; volume replacement – filling a defect with tissue from elsewhere (usually the latissimus dorsi muscle); and by surgery on the contralateral, normal breast to maintain symmetry using reduction mammoplasty techniques.

Breast reconstruction (Figure 3.10, 3.11)

All women undergoing mastectomy who are fit enough to undergo the procedure should be offered breast reconstruction. It is impossible to replace the breast but various surgical techniques can be used to create a breast mound which provides reasonable symmetry with the normal side when clothed and, ideally, naked. Unless the nipple has been preserved at the initial mastectomy procedure, it will be absent (but it can also be reconstructed). Reconstructed breasts have variable amounts of scarring and numbness. The reconstructed breast will also often not become ptotic with age particularly if an implant-based reconstruction has been used. Breast reconstruction can be performed at the time of mastectomy or at any time after oncological treatment is complete. There is no evidence that immediate reconstruction significantly delays subsequent adjuvant treatment but the adjuvant treatment (particularly radiotherapy) may affect the appearance and texture of the reconstructed breast and so affect selection of the type of reconstruction. It may not be possible to produce

symmetry at one operation but additional surgery can be performed on the contralateral normal breast either to reduce its size with breast reduction or to increase the size (augmentation) with an implant to achieve symmetry.

There are three commonly used techniques for breast reconstruction with multiple minor variations:

1 Implant/tissue expander-based reconstruction.
2 Latissimus dorsi flap reconstruction (with or without implant).
3 Lower abdominal flap reconstruction.

Radiotherapy (Figures 3.12–3.14)

Radiotherapy to the breast is required in most women following wide excision of breast cancer and reduces local recurrence rates to levels similar to those following mastectomy. Radiotherapy improves survival as well as reducing recurrence compared to wide excision alone. A dose of 40–50 Gy is given in fractions over 3–5 weeks as an outpatient procedure. The dose is given by external beam irradiation with careful planning to ensure that a predictable homogenous dose is delivered to the breast with as little irradiation of other structures as possible. Giving a further boost of 10–20 Gy locally to the tumour bed reduces local recurrence rates in women of all ages. As the absolute benefit is smaller in older women because local recurrence is less

3.12 The patient is carefully positioned at each attendance for radiotherapy to ensure consistent treatment. Laser beams are used to aid positioning. CT planning of the radiotherapy beams ensures the appropriate dose is given to the target area with as little irradiation of other structures as possible.

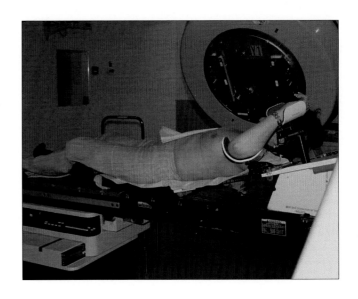

3.13 Forrest plots showing the proportional effects of radiotherapy following breast conservation therapy for breast cancer from a meta-analysis of 6 randomized trials in a total of 4177 women. Radiotherapy to the breast reduces local recurrence by about two-thirds (hazard ratio 0.32, p<0.00001). There is also a small reduction in breast cancer deaths (hazard ratio 0.86, p=0.04). Radiotherapy is, therefore, recommended for all patients following breast conservation surgery. (Adapted from Early Breast Cancer Trialists' Collaborative Group [2000], *Lancet* **355**:1757–70.)

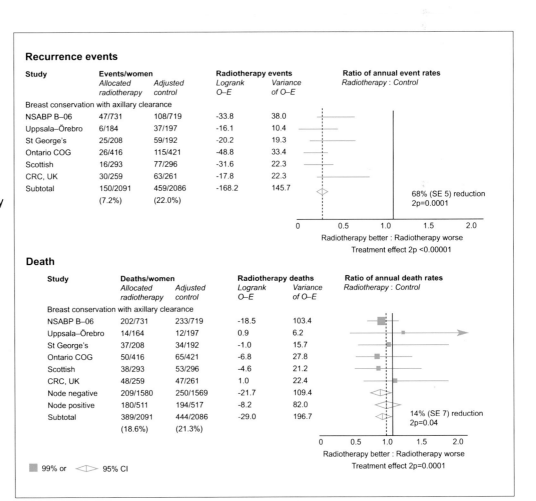

Recurrence events

| Study | Events/women | | Radiotherapy events | | |
	Allocated radiotherapy	Adjusted control	Logrank O–E	Variance of O–E	
Breast conservation with axillary clearance					
NSABP B–06	47/731	108/719	-33.8	38.0	
Uppsala–Örebro	6/184	37/197	-16.1	10.4	
St George's	25/208	59/192	-20.2	19.3	
Ontario COG	26/416	115/421	-48.8	33.4	
Scottish	16/293	77/296	-31.6	22.3	
CRC, UK	30/259	63/261	-17.8	22.3	
Subtotal	150/2091 (7.2%)	459/2086 (22.0%)	-168.2	145.7	

Ratio of annual event rates
Radiotherapy : Control

68% (SE 5) reduction
2p=0.0001

Radiotherapy better : Radiotherapy worse
Treatment effect 2p <0.00001

Death

| Study | Deaths/women | | Radiotherapy deaths | | |
	Allocated radiotherapy	Adjusted control	Logrank O–E	Variance of O–E	
Breast conservation with axillary clearance					
NSABP B–06	202/731	233/719	-18.5	103.4	
Uppsala–Örebro	14/164	12/197	0.9	6.2	
St George's	37/208	34/192	-1.0	15.7	
Ontario COG	50/416	65/421	-6.8	27.8	
Scottish	38/293	53/296	-4.6	21.2	
CRC, UK	48/259	47/261	1.0	22.4	
Node negative	209/1580	250/1569	-21.7	109.4	
Node positive	180/511	194/517	-8.2	82.0	
Subtotal	389/2091 (18.6%)	444/2086 (21.3%)	-29.0	196.7	

Ratio of annual death rates
Radiotherapy : Control

14% (SE 7) reduction
2p=0.04

Radiotherapy better : Radiotherapy worse
Treatment effect 2p=0.0001

■ 99% or ◁▷ 95% CI

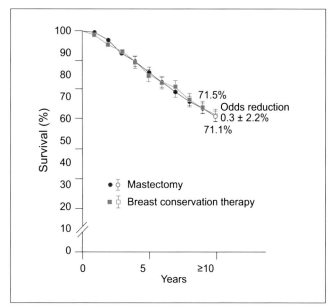

3.14 Overall survival curve prepared from meta-analysis of 7 randomized studies of a total of 3100 women with breast cancer treated with either mastectomy or breast conserving surgery plus radiotherapy. There is no difference in survival over more than 10 years and thus, when appropriate, breast conserving therapy by wide excision followed by radiotherapy to the breast is a safe alternative to mastectomy and preferable for the majority of patients. (Adapted from Early Breast Cancer Trialists' Collaborative Group [1995], *N Engl J Med* **333**:1444–55.)

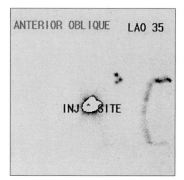

3.15 Lymphoscintigram following injection of technetium-labelled albumin (usually 20 MBq). A bright area is seen at the injection site and three 'hot' sentinel nodes are seen in the axilla.

common, many centres limit tumour bed boosting to younger women. Studies are under way to determine if local radiotherapy given just to the tumour bed and surrounding breast tissue will allow the omission of whole breast irradiation.

Radiotherapy is being increasingly used following mastectomy in those who have one or more factors that predict a higher rate of local recurrence such as muscle involvement, axillary lymph node involvement, lymphovascular invasion, a tumour size of more than 4 cm, and grade III tumours.

The provision of radiotherapy requires the patient to have reasonable arm mobility. Acute complications of radiotherapy include erythema and desquamation of the skin and tiredness. Subsequent healing following trauma, infection, or surgery in the irradiated area is impaired. Telangiectasia may be seen and tissues do not stretch as well after radiotherapy (which may limit options for reconstruction). Necrosis of skin and bone, pneumonitis, pulmonary fibrosis, and ischaemic heart disease, once regularly seen after radiotherapy, are now extremely rare.

Axilla

The axilla receives the majority of the lymphatic drainage from the breast. Up to 40% of breast cancer patients have involvement of axillary nodes by metastases at diagnosis. Axillary lymph node status has been consistently shown to be the most significant prognostic marker in patients with breast cancer. Evaluation of axillary lymph node status is therefore critical for accurately staging patients and provides a basis for making decisions on adjuvant treatment. If the axillary nodes arc not involved then no treatment to the axilla is required. If nodes are involved then treatment by surgical clearance or radiotherapy is required. Clinical and radiological prediction of lymph node involvement are not reliable but routine ultrasound scanning of the axilla followed by fine needle aspiration or core biopsy of suspicious nodes can confirm axillary node involvement in up to 40% of patients with positive nodes. In patients with invasive breast cancer without abnormal nodes on palpation or by ultrasound, a surgical procedure is required to assess axillary lymph node status. Lymphatic drainage occurs sequentially and the status of the first node draining the primary cancer indicates the nodal status of the regional lymph node basin. This first node is named the sentinel node (although in practice there are often 2–3 sentinel nodes). Procedures such as sentinel lymph node biopsy or an axillary node sample assess the status of the axillary nodes, but if the nodes removed are involved then subsequent axillary clearance or radiotherapy is required according to current protocols. Performing axillary clearance on all patients provides good staging information but provides no therapeutic benefit for node-negative patients and exposes them to the morbidity associated with this procedure and is not appropriate.

Lymph from perhaps 5% of the breast drains to the internal mammary nodes. Usually if the internal mammary nodes are involved there is also involvement of axillary nodes, but up to 1% of breast cancer patients have involved internal mammary nodes but no axillary involvement. It is possible, but not routine, to remove internal mammary

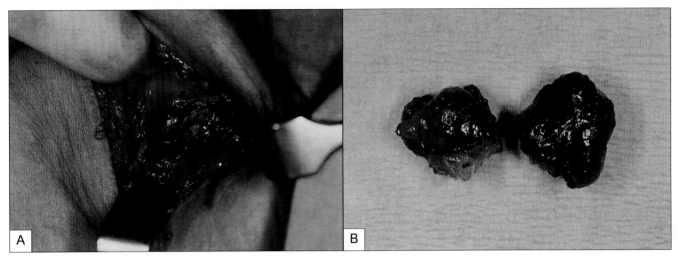

3.16A, B Injection of 1–2 ml of patent blue dye around the tumour or under the areola in the quadrant of the tumour allows the dye to be seen in the lymphatics leading to blue coloured sentinel nodes which can be sampled. Blue dye is often used in combination with radiolabel which helps in placing the incision and confirms that no residual sentinel nodes are present.

nodes (see below) but they are not always easy to remove and complications of removal include pneumothorax and intrathoracic bleeding. Underdiagnosis of involved internal mammary nodes rarely affects treatment decisions and failure to stage these nodes has not been shown to affect long-term outcome.

Axillary staging (Figures 3.15–3.17)

The majority of breast cancer patients do not have involved axillary nodes. Previously, axillary lymph node clearance was standard practice for patients undergoing surgery for early invasive breast cancer. The complications of axillary clearance and the increasing number of small screen detected cancers (with an overall node positivity rate of less than 25%) have driven the search for less aggressive axillary staging techniques.

The technique of four-node axillary sampling arose to exploit the relatively constant lymphatic drainage pattern and the fact that involved nodes were larger and thus easier to palpate. It involves making an incision over the lower axilla and excising at least four palpable nodes found on surgical exploration. Randomized studies in specialist centres have shown that in experienced hands four-node sampling does accurately predict axillary nodal status. The procedure is substantially quicker than axillary clearance surgery, results in less arm and shoulder morbidity, and can be performed as a day case. However, its use has remained restricted to a few centres.

The sentinel node biopsy technique has evolved to address the concerns of nontargeted four-node sampling by

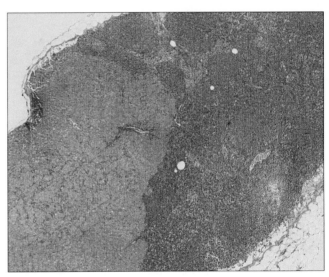

3.17 Replacement metastasis occupying the left side of the photograph of this axillary lymph node. H&E, original magnification x10.

providing a targeted and better defined nodal sampling technique. This involves the injection of blue dye and radiolabel into the affected breast prior to surgery. Traditionally, preoperative lymphoscintigraphy has been performed but this is probably not necessary. The use of an intraoperative gamma radiation-detection probe and visualization of blue dye in the nodes and lymphatics allows accurate sentinel node detection. This technique has been embraced with some enthusiasm. There remain some unanswered questions regarding the technique. The dose, colloid used, timing, and position of injection continue to be debated. The combination of blue dye and radiolabel increases detection of sentinel nodes but the blue dyes used have a significant risk of anaphylaxis (0.1–1%), blue dye may stain the skin for over 12 months, and use of radiolabel comes with substantial regulatory burdens. Using blue dye alone combined with lower axillary node sampling has the advantage that surgeons working in hospitals without a nuclear medicine facility can use this procedure although detection rates may be less than the combined technique. If the dye or radiolabel is injected around the tumour it can make surgery and localization awkward but sentinel internal mammary nodes may be identified.

Subareolar or intradermal injection is less messy and seems to identify axillary sentinel nodes successfully, but will not identify internal mammary sentinel nodes. If nodes are replaced by tumour cells they may not take up isotope or dye and can be missed if palpation for enlarged nodes is not also performed as in a four-node sample.

Axillary node involvement by metastatic disease on sentinel node biopsy or axillary sampling technique still requires definitive treatment by either surgical axillary clearance or radiotherapy. Techniques of intraoperative assessment of nodes have been explored, with touch imprint cytology and identification of tumour cells by molecular techniques having the highest sensitivity. They do require significant infrastructure to perform, they are not entirely reliable, and the patient and surgeon do not know what operation is to be performed prior to surgery, which can affect consent, planning of length of hospital stay, and operating list timing.

Advances in imaging and sentinel node technique offer the possibility of preoperative visualization and guided needle biopsy of one or more sentinel nodes to allow minimally invasive preoperative axillary staging.

Axillary treatment

The majority of patients with proven metastatic disease in axillary nodes are treated with surgical clearance of all axillary tissue up to the level of the axillary vein and to the medial edge of pectoralis minor (level 2) or to the apex of the axilla (level 3). The thoracodorsal pedicle to latissimus dorsi and long thoracic nerve to serratus anterior are preserved and intercostobrachial nerves should also be preserved if possible. Radiotherapy to the axilla and supraclavicular fossa is an alternative option if involved nodes are identified on an axillary sampling procedure. Drains are usually placed following surgery. Early arm mobilization with physiotherapy is encouraged.

Complications of surgery include bleeding, infection, and limitation of shoulder movement. Some numbness of the upper inner arm is common. Lymphoedema is the most feared complication of surgical axillary clearance, and causes troublesome problems in up to 10% of those following the procedure.

Recognition of the morbidity of the removal of all axillary nodes, and the fact that most breast cancer patients do not have apical axillary node involvement, has led to interest in limiting further axillary treatment if low volume disease is found at sentinel node biopsy. A recent study where no further axillary treatment was given to those with one or two positive sentinel nodes taken during conservation surgery has shown no obvious detriment and protocols for axillary treatment are being reexamined as a result.

SYSTEMIC TREATMENT OF EARLY BREAST CANCER

Treatment strategies

The majority of patients with localized breast cancer receive some form of systemic therapy. The intention of these systemic treatments (adjuvant therapy) is to kill or prevent growth of cancer cells which have escaped from the local area but have not yet grown to a size to cause local symptoms or be detectable on imaging. Systemic treatment can be given prior to local treatment (neoadjuvant therapy) which can also cause shrinkage of the primary tumour. This allows confirmation that the medication used is active against the cancer and may allow breast conservation for a lesion that would have been too large at diagnosis to allow this. The order in which systemic treatment is given does not appear to affect long-term survival. Three forms of systemic treatment are used: (1) hormonal therapy, (2) cytotoxic chemotherapy, and (3) immunotherapy directed against a specific tumour antigen.

Prognosis (Figures 3.18, 3.19)

It is not possible to predict precisely those who will develop recurrent or metastatic cancer and would therefore potentially benefit from adjuvant treatment and those who will not develop further disease who will thus not need treatment. An estimation of the risk of further problems can be gained using established prognostic factors. Factors known to be associated with increased risk of recurrence can be weighed together with issues such as general health to

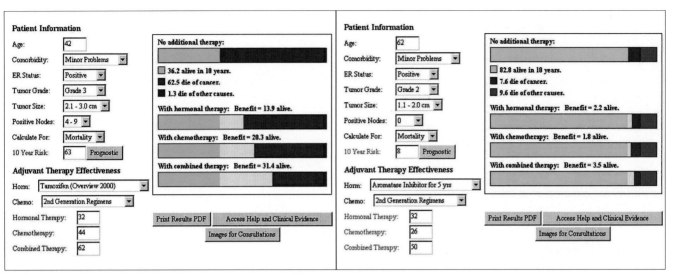

3.18 Internet-based resources, such as Adjuvantonline, offer estimates of patient outcome with or without various adjuvant treatments and can aid decision making by clinicians and patients. A patient with a fairly poor prognosis (**left**) has a reasonably large absolute benefit from adjuvant treatment while a patient with a good prognosis (**right**) has a little absolute benefit from adjuvant treatment although relative benefit may be similar. (Reproduced with permission.)

3.19 Graphical representation of expression of 70 genes from breast cancer specimens with relative up-regulation of gene shown as red and down-regulation as green. Those above the dotted line have a lower incidence of metastasis and appear to have different patterns of gene expression. Such gene profiles have been used to define high- and low-risk groups to aid decisions on adjuvant treatment. Traditional methods of prognostication result in treatment of a large proportion of patients, whereas this method may reduce the number of patients receiving apparently unnecessary treatment. (Source Van't Veer *et al.* [2002], *Nature* **415**:530–6 with permission.) (See *Table 3.1.*)

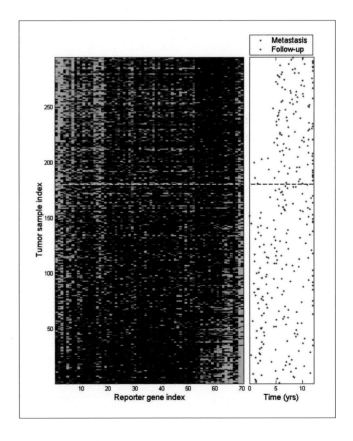

provide an estimate of the risk of recurrence and allow identification of those who have the most to gain by treatment.

It is important to recognize, however, that prognostication is an inexact science. Some patients deemed to be at low risk will develop recurrence, others at high risk who do receive treatment would not have gone on to have problems without treatment, and some at high risk who receive treatment will still die from metastatic disease. Importantly, these factors do not tell us who will gain benefit from treatment because

Table 3.1 Absolute versus relative benefit

- A relative survival benefit of 25% due to an intervention means that the chances of dying of the disease are reduced by 25%
- In a good prognosis cancer with survival without treatment of 90%, the chance of dying is 10% and so the benefit from the intervention is 25% of 10%, an absolute survival benefit of only 2.5%
- In a poor prognosis cancer with survival without treatment of 20%, the chance of dying is 80% and the benefit of the intervention is 25% of 80%, a much larger absolute survival benefit of 20%

Table 3.2 Nottingham Prognostic Index (NPI)

(0.2 x tumour size [cm]) + lymph node status (no nodes = 1, 1–3 nodes = 2, >3 nodes = 3) + histological grade (I–III)

Prognostic group	NPI Score	10-year survival without adjuvant therapy
Excellent	2.4 or less	94%
Good	2.4–3.4	83%
Moderate I	3.4–4.4	70%
Moderate II	4.4–5.4	51%
Poor	>5.4	19%

they are markers of increased risk not markers of benefit. These factors are used to try to balance known risks and side-effects that an individual will suffer against the potential benefit in terms of absolute chance of improvement or survival (*Table 3.1*).

Such risks and benefits inform the detailed discussions, initially within the multidisciplinary team and subsequently with each patient, to help arrive at the most appropriate treatment option for that individual. Tumour size, histological grade, receptor status, and axillary lymph node involvement together with patient age, menopausal status, and fitness are the main factors used to determine decisions on systemic therapy. Various tools exist to combine these factors and divide patients into groups according to risk including the Nottingham Prognostic Index (*Table 3.2*), St Gallen Consensus, and online tools such as Adjuvantonline. Analysis of genetic characteristics of individual cancers by systems, such as Oncotype Dx and Mammaprint, offers the prospect of more rational and tailored therapy and is beginning to be used to determine risk and guide treatment.

Hormonal therapy (Figures 3.20–3.24)

The response of a breast cancer to oophorectomy reported by Beatson from Glasgow in 1896 demonstrated that a reduction in oestrogen stimulation of breast cancer can cause tumour regression. While surgical ovarian ablation is used infrequently, medical ovarian suppression using an LHRH agonist is utilized in some premenopausal women in both the metastatic and adjuvant settings.

Tamoxifen is a selective oestrogen receptor modulator which has antagonistic actions in breast cancers bearing oestrogen receptors but agonist actions on endometrium, lipids, and bone. Tamoxifen reduces the risk of death from breast cancer by approximately 25% and is effective in all age groups regardless of menopausal status. A dose of 20 mg daily is usually given for 5 years. Tamoxifen reduces risk of contralateral breast cancer between 40 and 50% but may be less effective against human epidermal growth factor receptor (HER)2-positive tumours. It is more effective given after chemotherapy (if this is also indicated) rather than

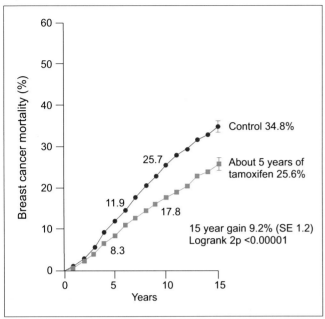

3.20 Graph showing the effect on breast cancer mortality of 5 years of tamoxifen treatment following local treatment of oestrogen receptor-positive (or unknown) breast cancer in 10,386 women. Breast cancer mortality is reduced by about one-third (hazard ratio 0.68, p<0.00001) and breast cancer recurrence is reduced by about 40% (hazard ratio 0.605, p<0.00001). This treatment was the standard of care for women with oestrogen receptor-positive breast cancer until the arrival of the current generation of aromatase inhibitors. (Adapted from Early Breast Cancer Trialists' Collaborative Group [2005], *Lancet* **365**:1687–717.)

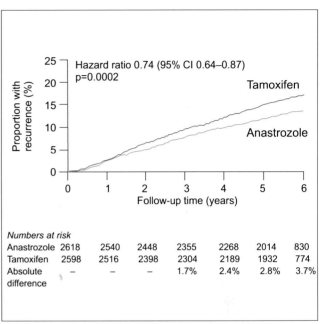

3.21 Graph showing the effect on recurrence of 5 years of treatment with anastrozole compared with tamoxifen following local treatment of oestrogen receptor-positive breast cancer in 6186 postmenopausal women in the ATAC study. Recurrence is reduced in those taking anastrozole by about one-quarter (hazard ratio 0.74, p=0.0002). There is no significant difference in overall survival (hazard ratio 0.97). (Adapted from Howell A, *et al.* [2005], *Lancet* **365**:60–2.)

concurrently. Side-effects include venous thrombo-embolism, hot flushes, gastrointestinal upset, vaginal discharge or dryness, altered libido, menstrual disturbance, and endometrial cancer.

Aromatase inhibitor drugs, which block conversion of androgens to oestrogens by the aromatase enzyme in postmenopausal women, markedly reduce circulating oestrogen concentrations. The currently available drugs include the nonsteroidal agents, anastrozole and letrozole, and the steroidal agent, exemestane. They are only effective in postmenopausal women with oestrogen receptor-positive tumours. Compared to tamoxifen, these drugs improve disease-free and metastasis-free survival in various settings but the situation is complicated by the fact that trials have used different drugs in different settings. They appear superior to adjuvant tamoxifen if given instead of tamoxifen (anastrozole and letrozole) or if patients are switched after 2–

3 years of tamoxifen (anastrozole and exemestane) compared with continuing on tamoxifen. Letrozole also reduces the risk of recurrence when used as extended adjuvant therapy after 5 years on tamoxifen. They reduce the risk of contralateral breast cancer by a further 40–50% above that achieved by tamoxifen. They also appear to be equally effective in both HER2-positive and negative cancers. Overall survival benefit has so far been demonstrated when used after 2–3 years of tamoxifen (switching) or after 5 years of tamoxifen (extended adjuvant).

Side-effects include hot flushes (less than tamoxifen), joint pain, osteoporosis, fatigue, and vaginal dryness. Aromatase inhibitors are more expensive than tamoxifen and many women require bone density monitoring during treatment because of the adverse effect of these agents on bone turnover. Recommendations are evolving constantly but it is suggested that very low-risk postmenopausal women are

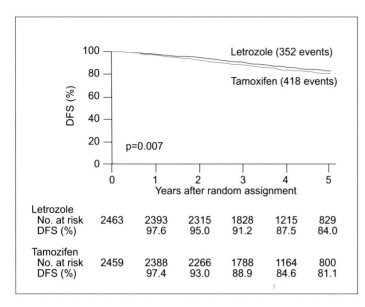

3.22 Graph of disease-free survival (DFS) following 5 years of treatment with letrozole compared with tamoxifen following local treatment of oestrogen receptor-positive breast cancer in 4922 postmenopausal women in the BIG 1-98 study. Recurrence is reduced in those taking letrozole by about 20% (hazard ratio 0.82, p=0.007). There is no difference in overall survival (hazard ratio 0.91). (Adapted from Coates AS, *et al.* [2007], *J Clin Oncol* **25**:486–92.)

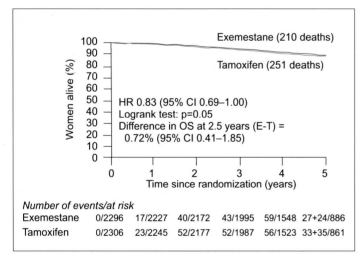

3.23 Graph of overall survival (OS) following 5 years of treatment with tamoxifen (T) compared with switching from tamoxifen to exemestane (E) after 2–3 years following local treatment of oestrogen receptor-positive breast cancer in 4724 postmenopausal women in the IES study. Switching to exemestane reduces mortality by about 20% (hazard ratio 0.83, p=0.05). Recurrence is reduced by one-quarter (hazard ratio 0.75, p=0.0001). (Adapted from Coombes RC, *et al.* [2007], *Lancet* **369**:559–70.)

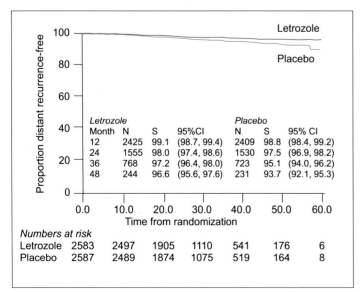

3.24 Graph of disease-free survival following 2–3 years of letrozole treatment compared with placebo following 5 years of treatment with tamoxifen following local treatment of oestrogen receptor-positive breast cancer in 5187 postmenopausal women in the MA.17 study. Recurrence is reduced in those taking letrozole by 40% (hazard ratio 0.58, p<0.001). There is no difference in overall survival (hazard ratio 0.82) although overall survival is significantly reduced in node-positive patients (hazard ratio 0.61, p=0.04) and those with tumours that are both oestrogen and progesterone receptor positive (hazard ratio 0.58). (Adapted from Goss PE, *et al.* [2005], *J Natl Cancer Inst* **97**:1262–71; Goss PE, *et al.* [2007], *J Clin Oncol* **25**:2006–11.)

treated with 5 years of tamoxifen, those at moderate risk take 2–3 years of tamoxifen followed by 2–3 years of an aromatase inhibitor or 5 years of tamoxifen followed by 3 years of an aromatase inhibitor, and those at high risk should receive 5 years of an aromatase inhibitor following surgical treatment.

Endocrine therapy can be used, particularly in postmenopausal women, as neoadjuvant treatment of large operable or locally advanced oestrogen receptor-positive breast cancers to reduce the size of cancers that are too large to allow breast conservation. The aromatase inhibitor letrozole achieves the best results in this setting and is the agent of choice.

In patients unfit or unwilling to undergo surgical treatment, endocrine therapy (letrozole in postmenopausal women) can be used either initially to permit surgery later or as sole treatment. Careful monitoring of such patients is required as tumours can escape from the control of endocrine agents even after months or years of response and then attention turns again to consideration of local therapy, often in less favourable circumstances.

Chemotherapy (Figures 3.25–3.29)

Cytotoxic chemotherapy uses drugs which kill dividing cells. The balance of efficacy and side-effects depends on the ability of a chemotherapy drug to kill cancer cells rather than normal cell populations which are turning over quickly. It is because these agents are poorly selective in their actions that side-effects are so common. A large number of agents are used in the treatment of breast cancer (*Table 3.3*). In the adjuvant setting, combinations of complementary agents are used to maximize the benefit of treatment. Formerly a standard treatment was CMF (cyclophosphamide, methotrexate and 5-fluorouracil) but this is now seldom used in isolation as anthracycline-based combinations (including drugs such as epirubicin and doxorubicin) have been demonstrated to be superior to CMF alone. Evidence is emerging that combinations of an anthracycline and a taxane (such as docetaxel and paclitaxel) offer further benefit above those of anthracycline regimens alone at the cost of increased rates of neutropaenic sepsis. High-dose regimens which

3.25 Chemotherapy (in this case epirubicin) being administered intravenously through an indwelling catheter.

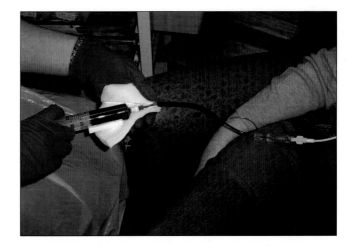

Table 3.3 Commonly used cytotoxic chemotherapy agents in localized breast cancer

	Type of agent	Particular side-effects	Common combinations
Cyclophosphamide (C)	Alkylating agent	Mucositis, cystitis	CMF, ECMF, FEC
Methotrexate (M)	Antimetabolite		CMF, ECMF
5-fluorouracil (F)	Antimetabolite		CMF, ECMF, FEC
Epirubicin (E)	Anthracycline	Cardiomyopathy, hair loss	ECMF, FEC
Doxorubicin (A)	Anthracycline	Cardiomyopathy, hair loss	AC
Docetaxel, Paclitaxel (T)	Taxane	Myelosuppression	ACT, FECT

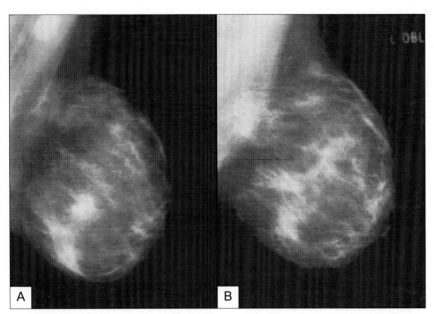

3.26 Mammograms showing response to 4 cycles of CMF chemotherapy (**A**: prechemotherapy; **B**: post-chemotherapy). The opacity in the breast due to the primary cancer, and that in the axilla due to a lymph node metastasis, have disappeared.

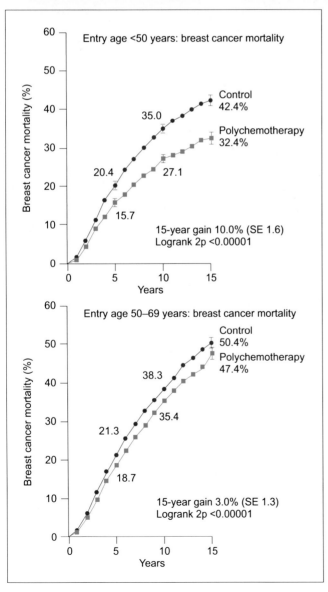

3.27 Graph showing the effect of polychemotherapy on breast cancer mortality following local treatment of breast cancer in those aged less than 50 (6974 women) and those between 50 and 69 (20476 women). Mortality is reduced with polychemotherapy but the degree of reduction is less with age (hazard ratio age <40=0.71, age 40–49=0.70, age 50–59=0.85 and age 60–69=0.91). (Adapted from Early Breast Cancer Trialists' Collaborative Group [2005], *Lancet* **365**:1687–1717.)

3.28 Graph of overall survival following chemotherapy treatment with epirubicin plus cyclophosphamide, methotrexate, and 5-fluorouracil (CMF) compared with CMF alone following local treatment of breast cancer in 2391 women in the NEAT/BR9601 trial. The addition of the anthracycline, epirubicin, reduced mortality by about 30% (hazard ratio 0.69, p<0.001). CMF is now rarely used alone and anthracyclines are utilized in the majority of those requiring chemotherapy. (Adapted from Poole CJ, *et al.* [2006], *N Engl J Med* **355**:1851–62.)

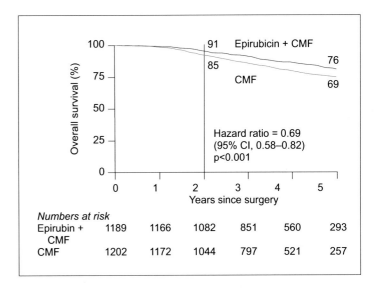

3.29 Graph of overall survival following chemotherapy treatment with docetaxel, doxorubicin, and cyclophosphamide compared with 5-fluorouracil, doxorubicin, and cyclophosphamide (TAC *vs.* FAC) following local treatment of node-positive breast cancer in 1491 women. The addition of the taxane, docetaxel, reduced mortality by 30% (hazard ratio 0.70, p=0.008). Taxanes are increasingly used as part of the chemotherapy treatment of those with high-risk breast cancer. (Adapted from Martin M, *et al.* [2005], *N Engl J Med* **352**:2302–13.)

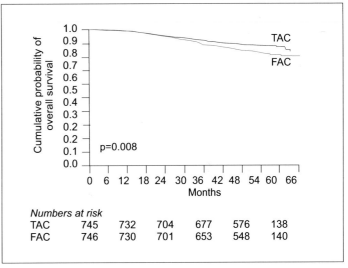

produce marrow ablation combined with autologous bone marrow or stem cell transplantation have shown no convincing benefit over more conventional regimens. Most agents are given intravenously for a finite number of courses (usually 6 or 8) every 3 or 4 weeks to allow recovery of normal tissues (mainly bone marrow). Recently, the use of medical stimulation of bone marrow recovery using granulocyte-colony stimulating factor (G-CSF) has allowed exploration of accelerated regimes with dosing every 2 weeks.

Common side-effects of chemotherapy include lethargy, nausea and vomiting, hair loss, mucositis, bone marrow suppression, and thromboembolism. Extravasation of chemotherapy agents can cause severe local tissue damage. Anthracyclines when given in large cumulative doses can cause cardiac damage and taxanes are associated with a high rate of neutropaenic sepsis and neurotoxicity. Because of the common and potentially serious side-effects of chemotherapy, its use is guided by expectation of benefit in

individual patients based on prognostication. Current anthracycline-based chemotherapy regimens offer an improvement in relative survival of around 35% in premenopausal women. This is reduced to 10–20% in older women.

Chemotherapy is commonly used in the adjuvant setting following local treatment of breast cancer in fit patients with moderate- and poor-prognosis cancers following discussion of the benefits and side-effects (*Tables 3.1, 3.4*). Endocrine therapy (which reduces turnover of cancer cells) is not generally used concurrently with chemotherapy (which kills cells turning over rapidly). Chemotherapy may also be used in the neoadjuvant setting for the initial treatment of localized large operable or locally advanced breast cancer, mainly in premenopausel women, in an attempt to reduce the size of the cancer or make it operable and to confirm activity of the agents against the individual cancer. This allows breast conservation in a proportion of patients but does not affect survival.

Table 3.4 Suggested adjuvant treatment following surgery for breast cancer

Risk category	Oestrogen receptor positive	Oestrogen receptor negative
Low risk Node negative, <2 cm, grade 1, >35 years, HER2-negative	Endocrine therapy or nil	Nil or chemotherapy
Intermediate risk Those not fulfilling criteria for low or high risk	Chemotherapy and endocrine therapy	Chemotherapy
High risk Node positive (unless 1–3 nodes only and HER2-negative)	Chemotherapy and endocrine therapy	Chemotherapy

Fitness and age may modify treatment recommendations. Endocrine therapy may be considered for oestrogen receptor-negative tumours that are strongly progesterone receptor-positive. (Based on Goldhirsch A, *et al.* [2005], *Ann Oncol* **16**:1569–83; Goldhirsch A, *et al.* [2006], *Ann Oncol* **17**:1772–6.)

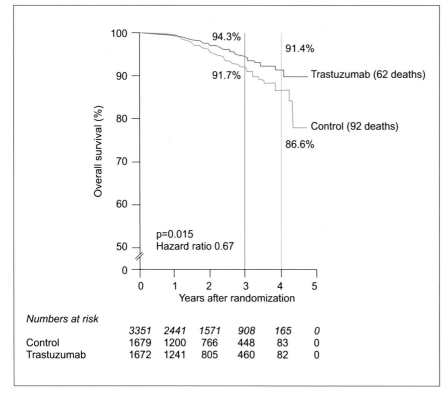

3.30 Graph of overall survival with or without treatment with trastuzumab for 1 year following local treatment for HER2-positive breast cancer and chemotherapy using doxorubicin, cyclophosphamide, and paclitaxel in 3351 women in the NSABBP B31/NCCTG N9831 trials. The addition of the HER2 receptor antibody, trastuzumab, reduced mortality by one-third (hazard ratio 0.67, p=0.015). Recurrence was halved (hazard ratio 0.48, p<0.0001). Trastuzumab is now widely used as part of the adjuvant therapy of those with HER2-positive breast cancer. (Adapted from Romond EH, *et al.* [2005], *N Engl J Med* **353**:1673–84.)

Immunotherapy (Figure 3.30)

A humanized monoclonal antibody to HER2 called trastuzumab has been developed. In patients with HER2-positive cancers administration of trastuzumab alone or in combination with cytotoxic chemotherapeutic agents improves survival in patients with metastatic disease and reduces recurrence when given in the adjuvant setting by approximately 50%. Because of its mode of action it does not have the side-effects of traditional chemotherapeutic agents but it can cause cardiotoxicity particularly when used in association with anthracyclines. It is costly and the appropriate length of a course of adjuvant treatment has not been established but is currently 12 months. It can also be very effective in the neoadjuvant setting in combination with chemotherapy. Patients who respond in the metastatic setting should continue on therapy at least until relapse, which may be some years.

The development of agents which bind a cytotoxic drug to trastuzumab may allow targeted delivery to tumour cells and minimize side effects. Other agents which target elements of the same pathway, such as lapatinib, pertuzumab and afatinib, are under investigation and show promise in the neoadjuvant and metastatic setting.

TREATMENT OF LOCALLY ADVANCED, METASTATIC AND RECURRENT BREAST CANCER

Locally advanced breast cancer (Figures 3.31, 3.32)

Locally advanced disease of the breast is characterized by features suggesting infiltration of the skin, dermal lymphatics, involvement of chest wall by tumour, or matted involved axillary nodes. The clinical features include:
- *Peau d'orange.*
- Erythema (skin inflammation).
- Direct skin involvement.
- Satellite nodules.
- Chest wall involvement.
- Fixed or matted axillary nodes.

Large operable breast cancers and resectable tumours fixed to muscle should not be considered as locally advanced. A cancer may be locally advanced because of:
- Biological aggressiveness (including inflammatory cancers).
- The position in the breast (for example, peripheral or superficial).
- As a consequence of neglect.

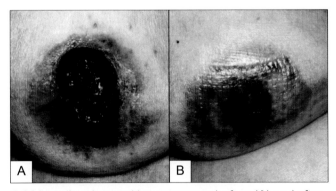

3.31 Locally advanced breast cancer before (**A**) and after (**B**) three months of treatment with letrozole showing a good response. A response to endocrine therapy like this may allow previously inoperable disease to become resectable.

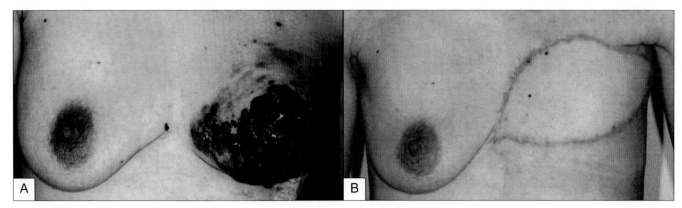

3.32A, B Latissimus dorsi flap for skin coverage. This patient presented with a locally advanced breast cancer with a large mass and multiple skin nodules. Following systemic therapy a mastectomy has been performed. The extent of disease required extensive skin resection leaving a wound which would not close primarily. To achieve skin closure and allow adequate resection, a latissimus dorsi myocutaneous flap has been performed.

Locally advanced breast cancers require multidisciplinary management. The patient's fitness and wishes are important in decision making.

Primary systemic therapy is often used initially in an attempt to downstage the tumour, which may allow such cancers to become operable. Conventional surgical resections are performed, most often mastectomy with axillary clearance, but breast conserving surgery is sometimes possible. Chemotherapy is preferred in the majority of fit patients (in combination with trastuzumab if HER2 positive) but endocrine therapy, usually with letrozole, is an option for postmenopausal women with oestrogen receptor-rich cancers. Following surgery, patients will usually receive radiotherapy either to the breast or to the chest wall, due to the high risk of recurrent disease in these cases. Local radiotherapy can be of particular use in those women with large areas of skin involvement and to control areas of cancer which are fungating or bleeding.

Surgical resection of large areas of skin and underlying tissue is sometimes performed in an attempt to completely excise locally advanced tumours, but the resulting defect may require coverage with a myocutaneous flap, and consideration should be given to the involvement of a plastic or thoracic surgeon in the treatment of such women.

There is a major contribution from neglect in many elderly patients where the cancers often behave in a rather indolent manner and may be well-controlled by endocrine therapy alone if surgery is not feasible due to general frailty.

Metastatic breast cancer (Figures 3.33–3.37)

The presence of metastases implies that breast cancer is no longer 'curable' but patients with metastases to certain sites may have minimal symptoms and survive for several years. In addition to a full clinical assessment of any specific symptoms and the patients' general health, an accurate knowledge of the site, number, and size of metastases is essential. To obtain this, imaging using plain radiology, ultrasound, computed tomography (CT), magnetic resonance imaging (MRI) and positron emission tomography (PET) may be required. Local treatment of the primary tumour or local recurrence if present is not usually performed unless local control is threatened, because any local disease can serve as an accessible measure of response to systemic therapy. Common sites for metastases include bone, lung, liver, and brain. Involvement of distant lymph nodes, ovaries, adrenals, and skin is also seen. Those with bony metastases alone may survive for several years while those with brain disease are likely to live only a matter of weeks.

Multidisciplinary team discussion forms the cornerstone of management planning for these patients. Endocrine therapy is given to those with oestrogen receptor-positive disease who are not immediately receiving chemotherapy. Aromatase inhibitors are usually used in postmenopausal women who have metastases at first presentation. In those that have previously received some form of endocrine therapy, an agent to which they have not previously been exposed is used. Those with bony metastases are usually prescribed bisphosphonates, which reduce bone turnover and slow progression of bony

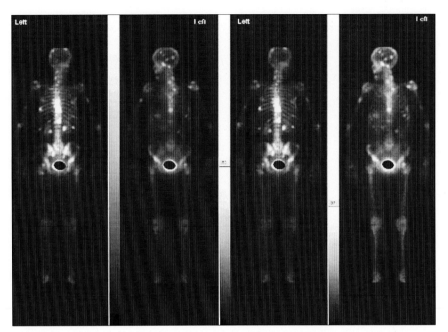

3.33 Bone scan images showing increased uptake of isotope in the skull, ribs, spine, pelvis, and humerus due to multiple bony breast cancer metastases.

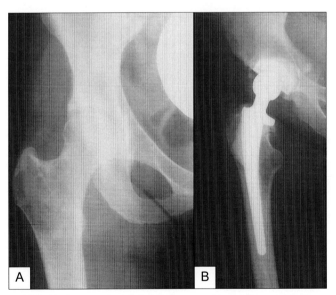

3.34A, B X-rays showing a lytic area in the femur due to destruction by a breast cancer metastasis. To prevent pathological fracture the femoral head has been replaced.

disease. Those with pain due to bony metastases usually have a good symptomatic response to a single dose of radiotherapy to the affected area. Risk of pathological fracture must be considered in those with long bone metastases and prophylactic internal fixation may be necessary.

Symptomatic patients with visceral metastases usually require chemotherapy. Similar agents are used to those in the adjuvant setting including trastuzumab, but additional agents

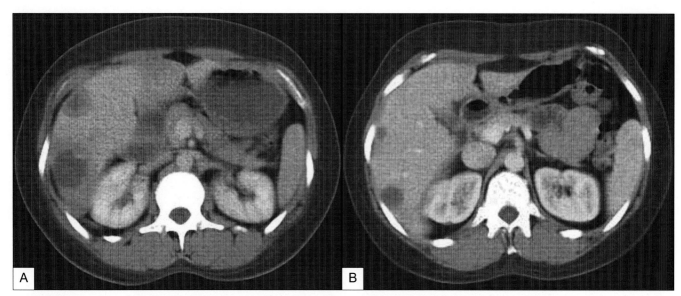

3.35A, B CT scans of the liver before and after 3 cycles of epirubicin chemotherapy showing marked reduction in size of liver metastases.

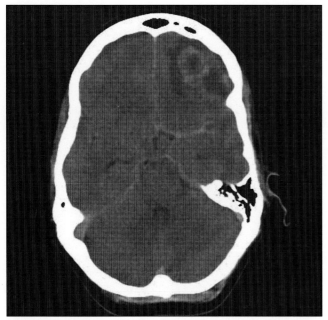

3.36 CT scan showing a lesion within the left frontal lobe with peripheral enhancement, surrounding oedema and some compression effects due to a breast cancer metastasis. This patient had other brain lesions and so was treated with steroids and radiotherapy. Single lesions in fit patients may occasionally be treated by excision.

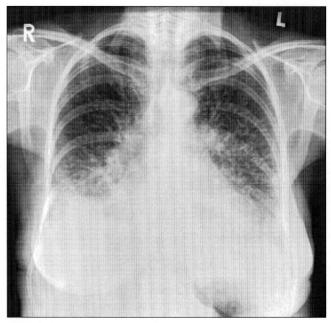

3.37 Diffuse patchy abnormality throughout both lung fields due to lymphangitis carcinomatosa from breast cancer.

including vinorelbine, capecitabine, and eribulin are sometimes used in the metastatic setting, particularly in women who have already been exposed to regimens including anthracyclines and taxanes. Irradiation and steroids can be useful in those with brain metastases. Involvement of palliative care specialists is often useful when therapeutic options are limited.

Specific problems seen in breast cancer patients with metastatic disease may require particular interventions. Hypercalcaemia is not uncommon in advanced untreated breast cancer, and usually develops as a result of bony metastases but can occur as a result of the release of parathyroid hormone-like substances by the cancer in women with no bony metastases. Hypercalcaemia can cause death due to cardiac effects and urgent treatment is required. Patients often have low albumin concentrations and therefore calcium concentrations need to be adjusted as an apparently normal calcium level can be significant. Treatment requires rapid rehydration and the administration of a bisphosphonate. Malignant pleural effusions are common and may require repeated drainage or pleuradhesis. Lymphangitis carcinomatosa is usually treated with steroids in combination with chemotherapy.

Spinal cord compression and superior vena cava obstruction require urgent radiotherapy. Management of pain will depend on its cause and specific interventions can be valuable. Use of the analgesic ladder is advised and the advice of pain teams and palliative care physicians is invaluable.

Recurrent breast cancer (Figures 3.38–3.40)

Breast cancer recurrence is feared greatly and affects as many as one-third of breast cancer patients in their lifetime. The aims of long-term review are to detect any treatable local recurrence or contralateral disease, to provide psychological support, and to address any problems associated with treatment. Women with a cancer in one breast have a 3 times relative risk compared to the general population of developing a cancer in the opposite breast. The risk is of the order of 6 per thousand per year. Regular mammographic follow-up of the contralateral breast, together with the involved breast if breast conserving surgery has been performed, is recommended. If recurrence is suspected, biopsy to assess the nature and hormonal receptor status is essential, as is a thorough assessment of any other disease at other sites. Approximately half of those with true local recurrence will also have distant metastatic disease.

Localized breast, chest wall, axillary disease, and accessible localized distant nodes may be treated by excision. This usually involves mastectomy if disease recurs within a treated breast. Endocrine therapy is usually changed or restarted in those with oestrogen receptor-positive disease, and radiotherapy is considered if recurrence is outwith a previously treated area. If the disease cannot be excised, consideration of treatment is according to the principles outlined for locally advanced disease. If distant metastases are present, treatment is as outlined for metastatic disease.

3.38 Mammogram showing a stellate opacity separate from the site of a previous breast cancer (marked by radio-opaque clips) due to a new or recurrent breast cancer. Mammographic follow-up detects many such lesions before they become palpable.

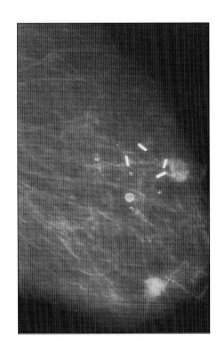

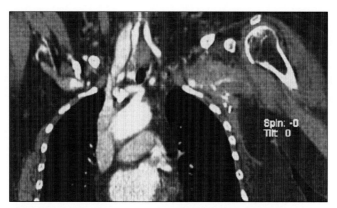

3.39 Reconstructed coronal contrast-enhanced CT scan image showing recurrence of breast cancer in the left supraclavicular fossa. A soft tissue mass is visible surrounding the axillary vessels. Surgical clips are visible towards the apex of the axilla from previous axillary clearance surgery.

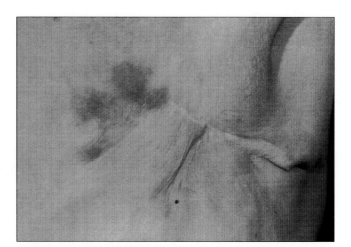

3.40 Recurrence following mastectomy for breast cancer. Several small discrete nodules of recurrent breast cancer are present on the chest wall. Small areas of skin recurrence without evidence of further metastases may be suitable for surgical excision.

Further Reading

CHAPTER 1: ANATOMY, PHYSIOLOGY, SYMPTOM ASSESSMENT, AND EPIDEMIOLOGY

Anatomy and physiology of the breast

Bland KI, Copeland EM (2009). *The Breast: Comprehensive Management of Benign and Malignant Disorders*, 4th edn. Saunders, St Louis.

JM Dixon (2012). *ABC of Breast Diseases*, 4th edn. BMJ Books, London.

JM Dixon (2009). *Breast Surgery. A Companion to Specialist Surgical Practice*, 4th edn. Elsevier, London.

Assessment of the breast

Bland KI, Copeland EM (2009). *The Breast: Comprehensive Management of Benign and Malignant Disorders*, 4th edn. Saunders, St Louis.

Dey P, *et al.* (2002). Costs and benefits of a one stop clinic compared with a dedicated breast clinic: randomised controlled trial. *Br Med J* **324**:507.

Eltahir A, *et al.* (1999). The accuracy of 'one-stop' diagnosis for 1110 patients presenting to a symptomatic clinic. *J Roy Coll Surg Edin* **44**:226–30.

Kuhl CK, *et al.* (2007). MRI for diagnosis of pure ductal carcinoma *in situ*: a prospective observational study. *Lancet* **370**:485–92.

Lehman CD, *et al.* (2007). MRI evaluation of the contralateral breast in women with recently diagnosed breast cancer. *N Engl J Med* **356**:1295–303.

Morris KT, *et al.* (2001). Usefulness of the triple test score for palpable breast masses. *Arch Surg* **136**:1008–13.

Turnbull L, *et al.* (2010). Comparative effectiveness of MRI in breast cancer (COMICE) trial: a randomised controlled trial. *Lancet* **375**:563–71.

Epidemiology of breast cancer

Beral V, *et al.* (2003). Breast cancer and hormone-replacement therapy in the Million Women Study. *Lancet* **362**:419–27.

Chlebowski RT, *et al.* (2003). Influence of estrogen plus progestin on breast cancer and mammography in healthy postmenopausal women: the Women's Health Initiative randomized trial. *JAMA* **289**:3243–53.

Claus EB, *et al.* (1994). Autosomal dominant inheritance of early-onset breast cancer. Implications for risk prediction. *Cancer* **73**:643–51.

Gail M, Rimer B (1998). Risk-based recommendations for mammographic screening for women in their forties. *J Clin Oncol* **16**:3105–14.

Garber JE, Offit K (2005). Hereditary cancer predisposition syndromes. *J Clin Oncol* **23**:276–92.

Hartmann LC, *et al.* (1999). Efficacy of bilateral prophylactic mastectomy in women with a family history of breast cancer. *N Engl J Med* **340**:77–84.

Jack RH, *et al.* (2009). Breast cancer incidence, stage, treatment and survival in ethnic groups in South East England. *Br J Cancer* **100**:545–50.

Meijers-Heijboer EJ (2001). Breast cancer after prophylactic bilateral mastectomy in women with a BRCA1 or BRCA2 mutation. *N Engl J Med* **345**:159–64.

Nelson HD, *et al.* (2009). Systematic review: comparative effectiveness of medications to reduce risk for primary breast cancer. *Ann Intern Med* **151**:703–15.

Rebbeck TR, *et al.* (2004). Bilateral prophylactic mastectomy reduces breast cancer risk in BRCA1 and BRCA2 mutation carriers. *J Clin Oncol* **22**:1055–62.

NICE (2006). Familial Breast Cancer. NICE Clinical Guideline 41, National Institute for Health and Clinical Excellence. London, www.nice.org.uk

Rossouw JE, et al. (2002). Risks and benefits of estrogen plus progestin in healthy postmenopausal women: principal results from the Women's Health Initiative randomized controlled trial. *JAMA* **288**:321–33.

Singletary SE (2003). Rating the risk factors for breast cancer. *Ann Surg* **237**:474–82.

Breast screening

Autier P, et al. (2011). Breast cancer mortality in neighbouring European countries with different levels of screening but similar access to treatment: trend analysis of WHO mortality database. *Br Med J* **343**:300.

Blanks RG, et al. (2000). Effects of NHS breast screening programme on mortality from breast cancer in England and Wales, 1990–1998: comparison of observed with predicted mortality. *Br Med J* **321**:665–9.

Kelager M, et al. (2010). Effect of screening mammography on breast-cancer mortality in Norway. *N Engl J Med* **363**:1203–10.

Kriege M, et al. (2004). Efficacy of MRI and mammography for breast-cancer screening in women with a familial or genetic predisposition. *N Engl J Med* **351**:427–37.

Moss SM, et al. (2006). Effect of mammographic screening from age 40 years on breast cancer mortality at 10 years' follow-up: a randomised controlled trial. *Lancet* **368**:2053–60.

Nystrom L, et al. (2002). Long-term effects of mammography screening: updated overview of the Swedish randomised trials. *Lancet* **359**:909–19.

Suhrke P, et al. (2011). Effect of mammography screening on surgical treatment for breast cancer in Norway: comparative analysis of cancer registry data. *Br Med J* **343**:d4692.

Tabar L, et al. (2003). Mammography service screening and mortality in breast cancer patients: 20-year follow-up before and after introduction of screening. *Lancet* **361**:1405–10.

www.cancerscreening.nhs.uk/breastscreen/index.html

CHAPTER 2: HISTOLOGY AND STAGING

Noninvasive malignancies and conditions of uncertain malignant potential

Bijker N, et al. (2006). Breast-conserving treatment with or without radiotherapy in ductal carcinoma *in situ*: ten-year results of European Organisation for Research and Treatment of Cancer randomised phase III trial 10853. *J Clin Oncol* **24**:3381–7.

Chuba PL, et al. (2005). Bilateral risk for subsequent breast cancer after lobular carcinoma *in situ*: analysis of surveillance, epidemiology, and end results data. *J Clin Oncol* **23**:5534–41.

Collins LC, et al. (2005). Outcome of patients with ductal carcinoma *in situ* untreated after diagnostic biopsy. *Cancer* **103**:1778–84.

Fisher B, et al. (1998). Lumpectomy and radiation therapy for the treatment of intraductal breast cancer: findings from National Surgical Adjuvant Breast and Bowel Project B-17. *J Clin Oncol* **16**:441–52.

Fisher B, et al. (1999). Tamoxifen in the treatment of intraductal breast cancer: National Surgical Adjuvant Breast and Bowel Project B-24 randomised controlled trial. *Lancet* **353**:1993–2000.

Houghton J, et al. (2003). Radiotherapy and tamoxifen in women with completely excised ductal carcinoma *in situ* of the breast in the UK, Australia, and New Zealand: randomised controlled trial. *Lancet* **362**:95–102.

Hussain M, Cunnick GH (2011). Management of lobular carcinoma in-situ and atypical lobular hyperplasia of the breast – a review. *EJSO* **37**:279–89.

Julien JP, et al. (2000). Radiotherapy in breast-conserving treatment for ductal carcinoma *in situ*: first results of the EORTC randomised phase III trial 10853. *Lancet* **355**:528–33.

Page DL, et al. (2003). Atypical lobular hyperplasia as a unilateral predictor of breast cancer risk: a retrospective cohort study. *Lancet* **361**:125–9.

Sanders ME, et al. (2005). The natural history of low-grade ductal carcinoma *in situ* of the breast in women treated by biopsy only revealed over 30 years of long-term follow-up. *Cancer* **103**:2481–4.

Silverstein MJ, et al. (1996). A prognostic index for ductal carcinoma *in situ* of the breast. *Cancer* **77**:2267–74.

Silverstein MJ, et al. (1999). The influence of margin width on local control of ductal carcinoma *in situ* of the breast. *N Engl J Med* **340**:1455–61.

Silverstein MJ, *et al.* (2003). The University of Southern California/Van Nuys Prognostic Index for ductal carcinoma *in situ* of the breast. *Am J Surg* **186**:337–43.

Smith BD, *et al.* (2006). Effectiveness of radiation therapy in older women with ductal carcinoma *in situ*. *J Natl Cancer Inst* **98**:1302–10.

Wapnir IL *et al.* (2011). Long-term outcomes of invasive ipsilateral breast tumor recurrences after lumpectomy in NSABP B-17 and B24 randomised clinical trials for DCIS. *J Natl Cancer Inst* **103**:478–88.

Histology of breast cancer

Harris JR, *et al.* (eds) (2009). *Diseases of the Breast*, 4th edn. Lippincott, Williams and Wilkins, Philadelphia.

Rosen PP (2008). *Rosen's Breast Pathology*, 3rd edn. Lippincott, Williams and Wilkins, Philadelphia.

Staging of breast cancer

Barrett T, *et al.* (2009). Radiological staging in breast cancer: which asymptomatic patients to image and how. *Br J Cancer* **100**:15228.

Baruah BP, *et al.* (2010). Axillary node staging by ultrasonography and fine-needle aspiration cytology in patients with breast cancer. *Br J Surgery* **97**:680–3.

CHAPTER 3: TREATMENT OF BREAST CANCER

Local treatment of early breast cancer

Arsalani-Zadeh R, *et al.* (2011). Evidence-based review of enhancing postoperative recovery after breast surgery. *Br J Surgery* **98**:181–96.

Association of Breast Surgery at BASO, BAPRAS and Training Interface group in Breast Surgery (2007). Oncoplastic breast surgery – a guide to good practice. *Eur J Surg Oncol* **33**:Suppl 1.

Avril A, *et al.* (2011). Phase III randomised equivalence trial of early breast cancer treatments with or without axillary clearance in post-menopausal patients results after 5 years of follow up. *EJSO* **37**:563–70.

Chetty U, *et al.* (2000). Management of the axilla in operable breast cancer treated by breast conservation: a randomised clinical trial. *Br J Surg* **87**:163–9.

Early Breast Cancer Trialists' Collaborative Group (1995). Effects of radiotherapy and surgery in early breast cancer: an overview of the randomized trials. *N Engl J Med* **333**:1444–55.

Early Breast Cancer Trialists' Collaborative Group (2000). Favourable and unfavourable effects on long-term survival of radiotherapy for early breast cancer: an overview of the randomised trials. *Lancet* **355**:1757–70.

Early Breast Cancer Trialists' Collaborative Group (2005). Effects of radiotherapy and of differences in the extent of surgery for early breast cancer on local recurrence and 15-year survival: an overview of the randomised trials. *Lancet* **366**:2087–106.

Early Breast Cancer Trialists' Collaborative Group (2011). Effect of radiotherapy after breast-conserving surgery on 10-year recurrence and 15-year breast cancer death: meta-analysis of individual patient data for 10801 women in 17 randomised trials. *Lancet* **378**:1707–16.

Fisher B, *et al.* (2002). Twenty-year follow-up of a randomized trial comparing total mastectomy, lumpectomy, and lumpectomy plus irradiation for the treatment of invasive breast cancer. *N Engl J Med* **347**:1233–41.

Fitoussi AD, *et al.* (2010). Oncoplastic surgery for breast cancer: analysis of 540 consecutive cases. *Plast Reconstr Sug* **125**:454–62.

Forrest APM, *et al.* (1995). The Edinburgh randomised trial of axillary sampling or axillary clearance after mastectomy. *Br J Surg* **82**:1504–8.

Giuliano AE, *et al.* (2011). Axillary dissection vs no axillary dissection in women with invasive breast cancer and sentinel node metastasis. *J Am Med Assoc* **305**:569–75.

Harcourt DM, *et al.* (2003). The psychological effect of mastectomy with or without breast reconstruction: a prospective, multicenter study. *Plast Reconstr Surg* **111**:1060–8.

Klough KB, *et al.* (2003). Oncoplastic techniques allow extensive resections for breast-conserving therapy of breast carcinomas. *Ann Surg* **237**:26–34.

Krag DN *et al.* (2007). Technical outcomes of sentinel-lymph-node resection and conventional axillary-lymph-node dissection in patients with clinically node-negative breast cancer: results from the NSABP B-32 randomised phase III trial. *Lancet Oncol* **8**:881–8.

Layfield DM, *et al.* (2011). Intraoperative assessment of sentinel lymph nodes in breast cancer. *Br J Surg* **98**:4-17.

McCulley SJ, *et al.* (2005). Planning and use of therapeutic mammoplasty: Nottingham approach. *Br J Plast Surg* **58**:889–901.

Mansel RE, *et al.* (2006). Randomized multicenter trial of sentinel node biopsy versus standard axillary treatment in operable breast cancer: the ALMANAC trial. *J Natl Cancer Inst* **98**:599–609.

Niewoehner CB, *et al.* (2008). Gynaecomastia and breast cancer in men. *Br Med J* 336:709–713.

Noguchi M (2008). Avoidance of axillary node dissection in selected patients with node-positive breast cancer. *Eur J Surg Oncol* **34**:129–134.

Rudenstam C-M, *et al.* (2006). Randomised trial comparing axillary clearance versus no axillary clearance in older patients with breast cancer: first results of International Breast Cancer Study Group Trial 10-93. *J Clin Oncol* **24**:337–44.

Vaidya JS, *et al.* (2010). Targeted intraoperative radiotherapy versus whole breast radiotherapy for breast cancer (TARGIT-A trial): an international, prospective, randomised, non-inferiority phase 3 trial. *Lancet* **376**:91–102.

Veronesi U, *et al.* (2002). Twenty-year follow-up of a randomized study comparing breast-conserving surgery with radical mastectomy for early breast cancer. *N Engl J Med* 347:1227–32.

Veronesi U, *et al.* (2006). Sentinel lymph-node biopsy as a staging procedure in breast cancer: update of a randomised controlled study. *Lancet Oncol* 7:983–90.

Systemic treatment of early breast cancer

BIG 1-98, (2009). Letrozole therapy alone or in sequence with tamoxifen in women with breast cancer. *N Engl J Med* **361**:766–76.

Buzdar A, *et al.* (2006). Defining the role of aromatase inhibitors in the adjuvant endocrine treatment of early breast cancer. *Curr Med Res Opin* **22**:1575–85.

Coates AS, *et al.* (2007). Five years of letrozole compared with tamoxifen as initial adjuvant therapy for postmenopausal women with endocrine-responsive breast cancer: update of study BIG 1-98. *J Clin Oncol* **25**:486–92.

Coombes RC, *et al.* (2004). A randomized trial of exemestane after two to three years of tamoxifen therapy in postmenopausal women with primary breast cancer. *N Engl J Med* 350:1081–92.

Coombes RC, *et al.* (2007). Survival and safety of exemestane versus tamoxifen after 2–3 years' tamoxifen treatment (Intergroup Exemestane Study): a randomised controlled trial. *Lancet* 369:559–70.

Cuzick J, *et al.* (2007). Use of luteinising-hormone-releasing hormone agonists as adjuvant treatment in premenopausal patients with hormone receptor-positive breast cancer: a meta-analysis of individual patient data from randomised adjuvant trials. *Lancet* **369**:1711–23.

Cuzick J, *et al.* (2010). Effect of anastrozole and tamoxifen as adjuvant treatment for early-stage breast cancer: 10-year analysis of the ATAC trial. *Lancet oncol* **11**:1135–41.

Early Breast Cancer Trialists' Collaborative Group (1998). Polychemotherapy for early breast cancer: an overview of the randomised trials. *Lancet* **352**:930–42.

Early Breast Cancer Trialists' Collaborative Group (2008). Adjuvant chemotherapy in oestrogen-receptor-poor breast cancer: patient-level meta-analysis of randomised trials. *Lancet* **371**:29–40.

Early Breast Cancer Trialists' Collaborative Group (2011). Relevance of breast cancer hormone receptors and other factors to the efficacy of adjuvant tamoxifen: patient-level meta-analysis of randomised trials. *Lancet* **378**:771–84.

Eiermann W, *et al.* (2001). Preoperative treatment of postmenopausal breast cancer patients with letrozole: a randomized double-blind multicenter study. *Ann Oncol* **12**:1527–32.

Galea MH, *et al.* (1992). The Nottingham Prognostic Index in primary breast cancer. *Breast Cancer Res Treatment* **22**:207–19.

Gianni L, *et al.* (2010). Neoadjuvant chemotherapy with trastuzumab followed by adjuvant trastuzumab versus neoadjuvant chemotherapy alone, in patients with HER2-positive locally advanced breast cancer (the NOAH trial): a randomised controlled superiority trial with a parallel HER2-negative cohort. *Lancet* **375**:377–84.

Goldhirsch, et al. (2011). Strategies for subtypes – dealing with the diversity of breast cancer: highlights of the St Gallen International Expert Consensus on the Primary Therapy of Early Breast Cancer 2011. *Ann Oncol* **22**:1736–47.

Goss PE, *et al.* (2005). Randomized trial of letrozole following tamoxifen as extended adjuvant therapy in receptor-positive breast cancer: updated findings from NCIC CTG MA. 17. *J Natl Cancer Inst* **97**:1262–71.

Goss PE, *et al.* (2007). Efficacy of letrozole extended adjuvant therapy according to estrogen receptor and progesterone receptor status of the primary tumor: National Cancer Institute of Canada Clinical Trials Group MA.17. *J Clin Oncol* **25**:2006–11.

Hickey M, *et al.* (2005). Management of menopausal symptoms in patients with breast cancer: an evidence-based approach. *Lancet Oncol* **6**:687–95.

Jakesz R, *et al.* (2005). Switching of postmenopausal women with endocrine-responsive early breast cancer to anastrozole after 2 years' adjuvant tamoxifen: combined results of ABCSG trial 8 and ARNO 95 trial. *Lancet* **366**:455–62.

Jonat W, *et al.* (2006). Effectiveness of switching from adjuvant tamoxifen to anastrozole in postmenopausal women with hormone-sensitive, early-stage breast cancer: a meta-analysis. *Lancet Oncol* **7**:991–6.

Levine MN, *et al.* (1998). Randomized trial of intensive cyclophosphamide, epirubicin, and fluorouracil chemotherapy compared with cyclophosphamide, methotrexate, and fluorouracil in premenopausal women with node-positive breast cancer. *J Clin Oncol* **16**:2651–8.

Martin M, *et al.* (2005). Adjuvant docetaxel for node-positive breast cancer. *N Engl J Med* **352**:2302–13.

Mauri D, *et al.* (2006). Survival with aromatase inhibitors and inactivators versus standard hormonal therapy in advanced breast cancer. *J Natl Cancer Inst* **98**:1285–91.

Paik S *et al.* (2004). A multigene assay to predict recurrence of tamoxifen-treated, node-negative breast cancer. *N Engl J Med* **351**:2817–26.

Piccart-Gebhart MJ, *et al.* (2005). Trastuzumab after adjuvant chemotherapy in HER2-positive breast cancer. *N Engl J Med* **353**:1659–72.

Poole CJ, *et al.* (2006). Epirubicin and cyclophosphamide, methotrexate, and fluorouracil as adjuvant therapy for early breast cancer. *N Engl J Med* **355**:1851–62.

Powles T, *et al.* (2002). Randomized, placebo-controlled trial of clodronate in patients with primary breast cancer. *J Clin Oncol* **20**:3219–24.

Romond EH, *et al.* (2005). Trastuzumab plus adjuvant chemotherapy for operable HER2-positive breast cancer. *N Engl J Med* **353**:1673–84.

Slamon DJ, *et al.* (2001). Use of chemotherapy plus a monoclonal antibody against HER2 for metastatic breast cancer that overexpresses HER2. *N Engl J Med* **344**:783–92.

Smith I, *et al.* (2007). 2-year follow-up of trastuzumab after adjuvant chemotherapy in HER2-positive breast cancer: a randomised controlled trial. *Lancet* **369**:29–36.

Thurlimann B, *et al.* (2005). A comparison of letrozole and tamoxifen in postmenopausal women with early breast cancer. *N Engl J Med* **353**:2747–57.

Van't Veer LJ, *et al.* (2002). Gene expression profiling predicts clinical outcome of breast cancer. *Nature* **415**:530–6.

www.cancer-math.net/brcancercalcs.html

Treatment of locally advanced, metastatic and recurrent breast cancer

Bonneterre J, *et al.* (2000). Anastrozole versus tamoxifen as first-line therapy for advanced breast cancer in 688 postmenopausal women: results of the tamoxifen or arimidex randomized group efficacy and tolerability study. *J Clin Oncol* **18**:3748–57.

Eiermann W, *et al.* (2001). Preoperative treatment of postmenopausal breast cancer patients with letrozole: a randomized double-blind multicenter study. *Ann Oncol* **12**:1527–32.

Gainford M, *et al.* (2005). Recent developments in bisphosphonates for patients with metastatic breast cancer. *Br Med J* **330**:769–73.

Management of breast cancer in women, SIGN Guideline 84 (2005). Scottish Intercollegiate Guidelines Network, Edinburgh. www.sign.ac.uk

Mauriac L, *et al.* (2003). Fulvestrant (Faslodex) versus anastrozole for the second-line treatment of advanced breast cancer in subgroups of postmenopausal women with visceral and non-visceral metastases: combined results from two multicentre trials. *Eur J Cancer* **39**:1228–33.

Mouridsen H, *et al.* (2001). Superior efficacy of letrozole versus tamoxifen as first-line therapy for postmenopausal women with advanced breast cancer. *J Clin Oncol* **19**:2596–606.

Mouridsen H, *et al.* (2003). Phase III study of letrozole versus tamoxifen as first-line therapy of advanced breast cancer in postmenopausal women: analysis of survival and update of efficacy from the International Letrozole Breast Cancer Group. *J Clin Oncol* **21**:2101–9.

Nabholtz JM, *et al.* (2000). Anastrozole is superior to tamoxifen as first-line therapy for advanced breast cancer in postmenopausal women: results of a North American multicenter randomized trial. *J Clin Oncol* **18**:3758–67.

Slamon DJ, *et al.* (2001). Use of chemotherapy plus a monoclonal antibody against HER2 for metastatic breast cancer that overexpresses HER2. *N Engl J Med* **344**:783–92.

GENERAL FURTHER READING

Association of Breast Surgery at Baso (2009). Surgical guidelines for the management of breast cancer. *Eur J Surg Oncol* **35**(Suppl 1):1–22. Available from: www.associationofbreastsurgery.org.uk

Breast Cancer (early and locally advanced) (2009). NICE Clinical Guideline 80.

Breast Cancer (advanced) (2009). NICE Clinical Guideline 81.

Management of breast cancer in women, SIGN Guideline 84 (2005). Scottish Intercollegiate Guidelines Network, Edinburgh. www.sign.ac.uk

Mansel RE, *et al.* (2009). *Benign Disorders and Diseases of the Breast*, 3rd edn. Saunders, London.

NCCN Clinical Practice guidelines in Oncology: Breast Cancer, National Comprehensive Cancer Network (2007). www.nccn.org

Sibbering M, Watkins R, Winstanley J, Patnick J, editors. Quality assurance guidelines for surgeons in breast cancer screening. 4th ed [internet]. Sheffield: NHS Cancer Screening Programmes, c.2009 [NHSBSP Publication No.20, updated 2009 Mar; cited 2011 Nov 28]. Available from: http://www.associationofbreastsurgery.org.uk.

Silva OE, Zurrida SE (eds) (2006). *Breast Cancer: A Practical Guide*, 3rd edn. Elsevier, Edinburgh.

Willett AM, Michell MJ, Lee MJR, editors. Best practice diagnostic guidelines for patients presenting with breast symptoms [internet]. London: Department of Health; c.2010 [updated 2010 Nov; cited 2011 Nov 28]. Available from: www.associationofbreastsurgery.org.uk.

Wishart GC, *et al.* (2010). PREDICT: a new UK prognostic model that predicts survival following surgery for invasive breast. *Breast Cancer Res* **12**(1): R1. [Internet resource available from: http://www.predict.nhs.uk].

www.adjuvantonline.com

www.breastcancer.org

www.breastpathology.info

www.cancerscreening.nhs.uk/breastscreen/index.html

www.library.nhs.uk/cancer

Index